MEDICALLY ASSISTED DYING

A Compassionate Alternative to Suicide

Revised Edition

Francis J. Clauss

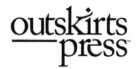

DEDICATION

To the ideals of our social and political system of democracy, as expressed by the Preamble to our Constitution ...

We. the People of the United States, in order to form a more perfect Union, establish Justice, insure Domestic Tranquility, provide for the Common Defense, promote the general Welfare, and secure the Blessings of Liberty to ourselves and our Posterity, do ordain and establish this Constitution for the United States of America.

... and to the political activists who work untiringly towards achieving those ideals.

PREFACE TO THE SECOND EDITION

While the chapter-by-chapter organization of the book remains the same, significant additions and changes have been made.

Chapter 1: Medically Assisted Dying as an End-of-Life Option, includes a note about the non-coverage for neurogenerative illnesses (e.g.. Alzheimer's, Parkinson's, Huntington's, and amyotrophic lateral sclerosis) in the Unit ed States.

Chapter 2: Experience of States with Medically Assisted Laws has been updated with results for medically assisted laws in Oregon and Colorado states to the end of 2018. It also includes information available at the time of writing for the challenge to overturn California's law for medically assisted dying. Chapter 2 ends with a discussion of the nationwide legalization of medical aid in dying across all of Canada implemented in 2016.

Chapter 3: Opposition to Medically Assisted Dying includes a discussion and rebuttal of a resolution of the 2017:2018 Congress of the United States against medically assisted dying. The Resolution includes an Introduction, 24 "Whereas" clauses, and the Resolution itself. A copy of the resolution itself is included in Appendix A with a detailed clause-by-clause rebuttal. The resolution provides a good summary in one place of what political opponents see as defects in the laws for medically assisted dying. Appendix A is essentially a misrepresentation of what suicide and medically assisted dying are, and the misuse of words to cause misunderstandings and biases that underlay the opposition.

It is significant that in the state and national elections of 2017 and 2018, most of the state and federal legislators who ran for office and had opposed medically assisted dying were defeated. Their defeats should encourage advocates who have been trying unsuccessfully to legalize medically assisted dying to continue their efforts, either by voter initiatives or by enactments by their state legislators.

The pope and bishops of the Roman Catholic Church remain in strong opposition to medically assisted dying. Despite the prelates' opposition, there is strong support among the Church laity in favor of medically assisted dying.

Chapter 4: Physicians and Healthcare Systems notes that the American Medical Association withdrew it opposition to medically assisted dying at its annual meeting in Chicago in June 2018 in favor of a neutral position while they restudy the issue.

Chapter 5: Healthcare, Patients, and Their End-of-Life Wishes has been rewritten and enlarged to include more information on the Affordable Care Act and other end-of-life options.

Medically assisted dying laws have been a great success in the seven states and District of Columbia where they have been made legal. The laws have enabled over 4,000 terminally ill patients to end their lives with compassion and dignity by ingesting a lethal medication at a time and under conditions of their own choice. The laws have restored sufficient autonomy to another 2,000 or more terminally ill patients who have continued to live and enjoy life, albeit limited by their illness and their other health and mental conditions, until they died from their terminal illness or some other intervening cause. For an unknown number of those who chose medically assisted dying, the laws provided a compassionate alternative to an ugly suicide

Medically assisted dying laws have also helped many thousands more family members and friends participate in the final hours of their beloved ones, and their experience has sustained them in their sorrow and shortened the period of their bereavement that followed.

Medically assisted dying laws have been a winning proposition for everyone involved.

Francis J. Clauss, Ph.D.
Palo Alto, California
March 25, 2019

PREFACE TO THE FIRST EDITION

Medically assisted dying is a compassionate alternative to a long and painful process of dying or to suicide. It bypasses life-support procedures and equipment that may be more objectionable than death itself. It allows individuals to end their lives with dignity — at times and under conditions of their own choice, typically surrounded by family and friends in a celebration of their lives.

Medically assisted dying was made legal by Oregon voters in 1998, twenty years ago. Since then, voters or legislators in six more states and the District of Columbia have enacted similar laws. Their legality has been confirmed by the United States Supreme Court.

During the past twenty years, more than three thousand terminally ill patients have used the medically assisted laws in the United States to die with dignity — on their own terms — rather than by ugly suicides.

* * * * *

My book is divided into five chapters. The first two deal with the codification of state laws for medically assisted dying, Chapter 1 describes what exactly medically assisted dying is, how it works to minimize pain and suffering, how it is controlled to prevent abuses, and how it differs from suicide and euthanasia.

Chapter 2 discusses the laws that have been enacted to legalize medically assisted dying. It begins with Oregon's Death with Dignity Act, which is followed by similar laws in six other states and the District of Colombia. The chapter discusses how the laws were enacted, how they have been opposed, how they have operated, and what they have achieved.

Chapter 3 discusses opposition to medically assisted dying, which is primarily due to prelates of the Roman Catholic Church and to misinformed or biased voters and legislators.

Chapters 4 and 5 discuss the physician and patient sides of the physician-patient interface. These are the focal points for implementing medically assisted dying and resolving any problems. Chapter 4 discusses changes in the medical profession to prepare physicians better for providing medical care for the elderly. It discusses some of the leading legal cases and court decisions that illustrate why we need laws for medically assisted dying.

Chapter 5 discusses the need for individuals to become more proactive in specifying how they wish to die and what types of healthcare they want to avoid. It summarizes the steps individuals need to take — from discussing their end-of-life wishes for dying with their doctors, their families, and their close friends to completing the legal forms used to document their wishes. It includes an overview of government programs that provide needed healthcare. It tells how to use a computer to obtain more information and to print copies of the forms used by various states, such as "Do Not Resuscitate" (DNR) orders and "Physicians' Orders for Life-Sustaining Treatment" (POLST).

* * * * *

Now step back from what you have just finished reading and recognize its impacts — that is, understand the revolutionary changes that are taking place in our healthcare system to implement medically assisted dying laws. Doctors, nurses, and medical scientists are shifting from being opponents against death to being limited partners with death. Sites for many dying patients have moved from hospitals to hospices and the homes of patients. Government agencies, from local to state and national, now regulate, oversee, and pay for armies of healthcare providers that are roughly as large and as costly as the combined total of our army, navy, and other military forces. The agencies levy and collect taxes and distribute what they collect to pay for operating the widely distributed components of our system for healthcare.

Courts of law, from state trial and appellate courts to the United States Supreme Court, are adjudicating conflicts between what is required, permitted, or denied to patients and their attending physicians. At the same time, they safeguard personal freedoms that are guaranteed to us by the Fourteenth Amendment of our Constitution.

Patients are themselves becoming more knowledgeable and vocal about the choices they can make under various scenarios of illness and accidents. They have become more proactive in working with doctors and other components of the healthcare system to satisfy their wishes for a compassionate and dignified death. Individuals are also becoming more active politically to enact laws for medically assisted dying and to defend such laws against attacks by opponents. Each of us plays an important role in this system.

* * * * *

My impetus for this book was twofold: First, it is a follow-on to my participation in the successful campaign to enact California's 2015 End-of-Life Options Act, which legalizes medically assisted dying for residents of the state. The campaign was ably led by the Compassion & Choices organization.

Second, my book is an attempt to respond to some controversial elements that are creating opposition to medically assisted dying. Those elements begin with misconceptions of what medically assisted dying is, what suicide is, and how they differ.

A personal note: After my father suffered a stroke that left him paralyzed on his left side and unable to talk, he was tethered against his will to life-support equipment that kept him alive. Under these conditions, he preferred death to living. When he attempted to use his right hand to pull the connections to the life-support equipment from his body, his right arm and hand were constrained. He was kept alive in this manner for nearly a year before being sedated to make him comfortable, disconnecting him from the life-support equipment, and allowing him finally to die.

I am very much in favor of medically assisted dying. I am proud to have been part of the efforts of many individuals, led by the Compassion & Choices organization, to enact California's End-of-Life Options Act in 2015 to make medically assisted dying legal for residents of California.

I acknowledge with thanks the help of my wife Mary Jean, my daughter Mary Ellen Clauss, RN, and friends Marrrilyn Stein, MD, Dee Standley, RN, Eleanor Swent, and Roberta Eidson for reading different versions of the manuscript and suggesting improvements. Any errors are, of course, the fault of the writer.

I hope that, after reading my book, you too will become an advocate to enact and defend medically assisted dying in your own state of residence. It is up to you to put your wishes for a peaceful death with dignity into action.

Francis J. Clauss, Ph.D.
Palo Alto, California
September 3, 2018

TABLE OF CONTENTS

PREFACE

Chapter 1

MEDICALLY ASSISTED DYING
AS AN END-OF-LIFE OPTION

"Grow old along with me! The best is yet to be.
The last of life, for which the first was made."[1]

In 2018, the life expectancy at birth of Americans of all races and both sexes was 78.7 years. For comparison, in 1900, a little more than a century ago, it had been only 47.3 years.[2] And worldwide that same year, the life expectancy at birth had been only 31 years! The increase in life expectancy is certainly something that is basically good.

In 1932, at the time the life expectancy of Americans at birth had climbed to around 60, a self-help book titled *Life Begins at Forty*[3] was published that was very popular and influential. Written by the American psychologist Walter Pitkin, it was the number one best-selling non-fiction book in the United States in 1933 and number two in 1934. The book's title became an American catchphrase, the title of a 1935 movie starring Will Rogers, a 1937 song sung by Sophie Tucker, and a 1980 song by the Beatle John Lennon. The book's optimistic view was that by maintaining a positive attitude, we could all look forward to many years of a happy, fulfilling existence after reaching the age of 40, followed by a blissful semi-retirement that was free from hard work and the responsibilities of childcare.

We owe much of the increase in our life expectancy to better nutrition, more active life styles, and better sanitation. More is due to vaccines and antibiotics developed by medical science. Vaccines prevent or ameliorate infectious diseases caused by viruses, such as chickenpox, hepatitis A and B, influenza, measles, mumps, poliomyelitis, and smallpox. Antibiotics such as penicillin and sulfonamides help prevent infections caused by bacteria. Still more increases in life expectancy come from improved techniques for detecting and treating various illnesses, and from better care provided by physicians, nurses, hospitals and other healthcare facilities.

Most importantly, our increased life expectancy is largely due to the availability of healthcare services and medicines as part of the public healthcare provided by our federal government. Major advances in federal programs for healthcare began with the Public

Health Service Act of 1944, continued with the Medicare and Medicaid programs of 1966, and reached a culminating goal of universal healthcare to citizens of the United States with the Patient Protection and Affordable Care Act (PPACA), often shortened to the Affordable Care Act (ACA) and nicknamed Obamacare. ACA was signed into law by President Barack Obama on March 23. 2010. Federal support also includes the sponsorship of medical research at various hospitals, schools of medicine, and government agencies. (See Chapter 5 for a short history of federal involvement in health-care for individuals.)

But while the increase in our lifetimes has been basically good, it has not been *all* good. Although the hopes for "life after forty" have been largely realized, they are offset by some of the realities of growing older. These became manifest in the second half of the 20th century. They showed up in jumps in the rates for depression and suicide in the latter part of the 1900s.

Suicide rates are measured by the number of people who commit suicide per 100,000 population, which takes into account changes in the population size. According to data from the National Center for Health Statistics, over the past 47 years for which data is available, the annual suicide rate in the United States has increased from 10.5 per 100,000 in 1969 to 13.0 per 100,000 in 2016. This was an increase of 24 percent. For adults aged 75 years or more, the jump was somewhat higher than for the overall population. Depression over such issues as the loss of personal autonomy, the enjoyment of life, and the control of body functions accounts for over 50 percent of those who died by suicide. If the number of depressed individuals includes those who sought relief by alcoholism, that number increases to 75 percent.

We are most grateful for the longer lives many of us enjoy. However, many are distressed by the onset of various types of cancer that are incurable and painful:
- by blindness or deafness that makes reading, watching television, or conversation difficult or impossible;
- by the loss of balance that causes falls and broken bones that limit mobility;
- by the loss of ability to drive an automobile;
- by a variety of chronic illnesses that leave us bedridden;
- or by the loss of control over essential body functions.

These conditions, often in combination, are making life's end painful and devastating for many individuals, their families, and their friends.

And, with advancing age, medical treatments may simply delay death without alleviating illness or pain.

As Dr. John P. Geyman, a physician with many years of experience treating terminally ill patients reported: "With advancing medical technology, many patients are subject to active and ineffective therapeutic efforts by their physicians, even when an early terminal outcome is not in doubt. As a result, many experience prolonged deaths often involving pain, suffering and loss of dignity. In reaction to this problem, an increasing number of patients want more direct control over the type of care they receive in the last stage of their lives."[4]

Others experience agonizing pain or are fearful of its onset as they continue to age. They wish to shorten the process of dying and avoid a lingering death and its associated pain, loss of autonomy or control of their lives, and an inability to enjoy life

During the latter half of the twentieth century, a great deal of attention was given to euthanasia (aka also known as mercy killing), to medical ethics, and to legal issues of end-of-life healthcare and its options. The last can restore some control to terminally ill patients over the process of dying and are classed as medically assisted dying (MAD) or medical aid in dying (MAID) laws.

Unfortunately, MAD and MAID are also called a form of suicide, such as assisted suicide or physician-assisted suicide. Such names are *incorrect, biased, and confusing.* Medically assisted dying or medical aid in dying have nothing to do with committing suicide, and it is wrong and misleading to imply they do.

In 1998, Oregon state's Death with Dignity Act made Oregon the first of the United States with a law that allowed medically assisted dying. Since then, six other states (Washington, Vermont, Colorado, Montana, California, and Hawaii) plus the District of Columbia have also enacted medically assisted dying laws modeled after Oregon's. Voter initiatives and legislative actions are underway in additional states to legalize medically assisted dying.

This chapter describes what medically assisted dying is, how it works, how it is controlled to prevent abuses, and how it differs from suicide, assisted suicide, euthanasia, and physician-assisted suicide. Chapter 2, which follows this chapter, recounts experiences and successes to date with the state laws currently in effect for medically assisted dying, and Chapter 3 discusses the opposition to initiatives and legislation action to enact medically assisted dying laws in additional states. The final two chapters discuss the implementation of medically assisted dying laws – Chapter 4 from the standpoint of doctors and lawyers, and Chapter 5 (which is the final chapter) from the standpoint of patients and the healthcare system. Chapter 5 includes brief descriptions of the Medicare and Medicaid programs of 1966, the Affordable Care Act of 2010, and other federal healthcare programs.

MEDICALLY ASSISTED DYING LAWS

For some, a longer life is a blessing. For many others, it's a curse.

Each of us wishes for a "good death" at the end of our life. We fear a "bad death" of becoming useless, demented, incontinent, in severe and continual pain, with poor eyesight and hearing, unable to walk, and dependent on others. We want some control over our dying, with our dignity intact. We do not want medical care that tethers us to life-support equipment or treatments that feel worse than death itself. We assert our constitutional right, guaranteed by the Fourteenth Amendment, to reject all forms of healthcare or life-support we do not want to receive or continue. Beyond those wishes, we would welcome being able to use medical means to restore our autonomy and self-control and to avoid pain.

Medically assisted dying (MAD) or medical aid in dying (MAID) laws address such wishes.

They are a response to some unwanted consequences of modern medicine's prolonging the process of dying. They are intended to restore the autonomy of terminally ill patients over their lives and their bodies. They give terminally ill patients some control over the conditions and progress of dying as well as the final act of death itself. They provide a compassionate alternative to suicide that allows terminally ill patients to die with dignity. In short, medically assisted dying laws permit patients themselves to decide how and when they will die. They allow terminally ill patients to choose the times, conditions, and settings for their deaths.

Medically assisted dying laws respect the final wishes of terminally ill patients. Their intent is to end a long and distressing period that often precedes death and can only end by dying. They end a patient's agonies during their final days or months. They typically end in a celebration of life, with family members and close friends gathered together and embracing one another in an edifying expression of love and the beauty of life. They are a compassionate alternative to suffering or to death by suicide.

The laws for medically assisted dying have been enacted by voters, either directly by voter initiatives or indirectly through their elected state legislators, who act on their behalf as part of our social and political system of democracy.

To date (March 2019), state laws for medically assisted dying have permitted more than four thousand terminally ill patients in the United States to choose the dates, times and conditions for ending their lives with dignity. The enactment, opposition, implementation, operation, and success of these laws are summarized in Chapter 2.

Terms and Acronyms

Medically assisted dying (MAD) is also correctly and commonly known by such description terms and acronyms as medical aid in dying. Other terms are physician assisted dying (PAD), and death with dignity (DWD), as well as physician-assisted death, aid in dying, dying with dignity, compassionate death, compassionate dying, medical assistance at the end of life, and a few other terms. The different terms place emphasis on various elements or characteristics of the law.

There are also terms that, though commonly used, are incorrect and misleading, such as assisted suicide, euthanasia, and physician-assisted suicide.

The three words in the term "medically assisted dying" are descriptive and accurate for what takes place.

- The subject of the matter is "dying." Using "dying" emphasizes that the focus of medically-assisted dying laws is on the process of dying rather than its end, which is death. The mentally competent adults who have access to the laws have already been diagnosed as having begun the process of dying, with a prognosis that it will end in six months or less. The law restores some of their autonomy and control over the conditions and duration of their dying. It allows them to choose the time and setting when they themselves will end their dying by ingesting a lethal drug, typically in their own home surrounded by family and friends for a celebration of their lives and a final goodbye — a death with dignity and compassion.

For those who choose to end their lives by medically assisted dying, their choice is not between living and dying because living is no longer a choice — they have a prognosis of not more than six months to live, and their real choice is how they will spend their final period of dying and when and how they will finally die.

Two-thirds of those who receive lethal drugs under a medically assisted dying law ingest their lethal dose and die well within the six months of their prognosis, with a median time of eight weeks after receiving the lethal dose. The other one-third of those who receive lethal drugs have enough of their autonomy and control over their lives restored that they choose *not* to ingest their lethal drug but *continue to live* — albeit under the conditions of dying. Most of them die of their underlying illness within their six months prognosis, others die between six months and a year from receiving the lethal dose, and a few have continued to live for more than two years before finally dying.

- The term "assisted" indicates that the roles of all participants, other than terminally ill patients themselves, are as assistants to the patients. As specified in the laws that have legalized it, MAD involves several individuals in addition to a terminally ill patient — two doctors, possibly a psychologist or psychiatrist, a pharmacist, and two witnesses to the patient's signing a form to allow the procedure. Each of these individuals acts as an assistant to help terminally ill patients obtain a lethal drug. The final act of ingesting the lethal drug is done by the patients themselves, without further assistance from anyone else.

   No individual is singled out by the term "medically assisted dying," and each assistant and terminally ill patient participates by choice rather than through coercion. The laws protect each from being charged with wrongdoing, provided they act in accordance with the laws' provisions.

- The term "medically" indicates that MAD is a medical process. It involves different parts of the healthcare system.

   The role of the first or attending physician is essentially to make sure that the patient using the law to end their dying is a competent adult (or is represented by a legal surrogate), is terminally ill, understands the alternatives to their choice of medically assisted dying (e.g., hospice care, pain palliation, and refusal or withdrawal of life-support care), and that the law's provisions are all carried out properly, without abuse or misuse. The second or consulting physician's role is to verify that the acts of the first or attending physician are in full compliance with the law's requirements.

The lethal drug and the pharmacist who provides it are other essential components of the healthcare or medical system. So is the government healthcare agency that regulates, oversees, and pays much of the costs for implementing medically assisted dying. Just as medical science and healthcare have added years of expected life at the birth of an individual, so is the system used to shorten the final months of their dying. More is said of the systems approach and it components in the chapters that follow.

Medically assisted dying is a term that removes the bias associated with such terms as suicide and death. It is a neutral term that helps make discussions between physicians and their patients easier and more meaningful. It facilitates rather than discourages discussions about end-of-life options between terminally ill patients and their families. It prepares families and friends for the impending deaths of their loved ones, and it helps them accept the inevitable. Studies show that the families who have had terminally ill members end their lives by means of medically assisted dying do not suffer as much bereavement from their loss as do those who have witnessed a family member or friend die an agonizing death.

Protection against Potential Misuse or Abuse

State laws for medically assisted dying define specific step-by-step procedures and conditions for obtaining and using a lethal drug. The procedures and conditions have been designed to prevent abuses or misuses of the laws. They must be followed "to the letter" by patients, their physicians, pharmacists, healthcare facilities, and any others involved in the procedure. Criminal action may follow if any step in the procedures does not fully adhere to the law.

Oregon's voter-enacted Death with Dignity Act (DWDA) of 1998 and others modeled after it typically impose provisos or caveats such as the following:

- The patient must be an adult (18 or over) and a resident of the state in which medically assisted dying has been legalized.
- The patient must be terminally ill, which means they have been diagnosed as having less than six months to live, as determined by two physicians.
- The patient must be mentally competent, verified either by two physicians or by referral to a mental health organization for evaluation. The patient's wish to die must be a rational choice,

considering the patient's condition and circumstance. The wish to die must not be because the patient is depressed, for example, and the patient's circumstances should be free of undue influence or coercion by others, such as manipulation by family members stressed by prolonged care of the patient or the urging of an heir to the patient's estate.

If either physician believes the patient is not mentally competent to make an informed decision for medically assisted dying, or if either feels the patient's request may be motivated by depression or another's coercion, they must refer the patient to a psychologist or psychiatrist. (Roughly 5 percent of patients requesting medically-assisted dying have been referred for mental evaluation.)

- The patient must be examined by two physicians, an attending physician and a consulting physician. The two will consult together on the patient's condition and confirm the patient's diagnosis and prognosis for the patient's dying within six months from their illness. One of the two physicians will prescribe the lethal medication. The attending physician also helps the patient navigate through the administrative details and paperwork that are safeguards to protect patients and prevent abuses.

- The doctors must inform the patient of all other options including hospice or comfort care, palliative care (aka pain control), care for depression, and their right to use voluntarily stopping eating and drinking (VSED) to end their life. They must also inform the patient that they can change their minds at any time. A significant percentage of terminally ill patients who initiate the process for medically assisted dying do change their minds at this point. Instead of asking for the lethal medication to complete their dying process, they choose hospice care, pain palliation, or care for depression.

- The patient must make two requests for a lethal prescription at least 15 days apart. The first is oral, and the second is both oral and in writing. The requests must be voluntary, made without coercion, verified by two physicians, and confirmed by two witnesses. At least one of the two witnesses must not be related to the patient, must not be entitled to any portion of the patient's estate, must not be the patient's physician, and must not be employed by the health care facility caring for the patient. No one present should coerce or unduly influence the patient's request for medically assisted dying.

- The written request must be witnessed and signed by two independent witnesses, at least one of whom is not related to the patient or employed by the health care facility.
- There is a 48-hour waiting period between the patient's written request and the physician's writing a prescription for the lethal drug.
- The attending physician should encourage the patient to discuss their decision, including their request for a lethal drug, with family members or next-of-kin. (This is not required because of confidentiality laws,)
- The patient may change or rescind their request at any time. The attending physician must offer the patient an opportunity to rescind their request at the end of the 15-day waiting period following the initial request to participate.
- The attending physician must certify that the patient's cause of death listed on the death certificate is the terminal illness or condition that had been diagnosed as likely to cause death in six months or less from the time of diagnosis, or to another cause that intervened.
- The primary function of medically assisted dying laws is to protect physicians from legal liability for aiding, assisting, or encouraging another to take their life, which under normal conditions is a crime. By conforming to the conditions of the law, physicians are protected from liability for prescribing a lethal medication for a terminally ill, competent adult.
- By conforming to the conditions of the law, the patient's decision to end their life does not affect the provisions of a life, health, or accident insurance or annuity policy, and the cause of death is recorded on their death certificate as their terminal illness, or a different condition that has intervened to cause death, or as "natural causes."
- Each physician (and the psychiatrist or psychologist, if one was used) should document their evaluations of a patient's health, mental condition, and their prognosis.

Physicians and others who participate in medically assisted dying are protected from criminal liability only in states that have legalized it and only when the physicians have followed specific procedures or caveats — that is, with legal warnings, specific stipulations, conditions, or limitations that have been defined by law and must be complied with. These caveats are designed to protect from prosecution the physicians who prescribe lethal drugs in accordance with the laws, pharmacists who provide the prescribed legal doses, and others who give assistance, as well as to protect terminally ill patients from potential abuses of the laws for medically assisted dying.

Unless protected by a state law that legalizes medically assisted dying, anyone who aids, assists or encourages another to take their own life may be prosecuted as a criminal.

Using Lethal Drugs to End the Dying Process

The final act of medically assisted dying takes place by the unaided ingestion of a lethal drug by a terminally ill patient that puts an end to the process of dying.

To prepare for the ingestion of the lethal dose, the patient should not consume fatty foods for four to six hours before the process of dying begins. It is best to take the lethal drug on an empty stomach to increase the rate of its absorption. The recommended procedure that follows has three steps:

- First, to prevent nausea, gagging or vomiting later, when ingesting the lethal dose, the patient takes an antiemetic such as metoclopramide or ondansetron.
- Second, the lethal dose is prepared by mixing 9 grams of a short-acting barbiturate, such as secobarbital (59.3% of patients), pentobarbital (34.3%), phenobarbital (5.0%), or other, such as a combination of the three named barbiturates and/or morphine (1.5%), in a half cup of water.

Secobarbital (aka seconal) was the barbiturate most commonly used when Oregon's law went into effect in 1998. A dose then cost about $150. In February 2015, after the Canadian drug-maker Valeant Pharmaceuticals International acquired it, the price of a lethal (10-gram) dose of seconal went up to $1,500 retail. It has since doubled. Alternative medications have been developed that are available at lower cost. One is known as DDMP, short for a mix of diazepam (aka Valium), digoxin, morphine and propranolol. A dose costs between $300 and $600. and it is reportedly being used in Washington and California.[5] Some pharmacies may prepare the mix into a slurry for the patient to ingest.

Under current law, federal funds cannot be used to pay for medically assisted dying. Patients should contact their insurers to determine whether or not their policies cover any of the costs of medically assisted dying. State laws vary, and to avoid any appearance of coercion, insurance companies cannot initiate informing patients that they will provide coverage for lethal drugs or other costs of medically assisted dying.

• Third, 45 minutes to an hour after the first step, the patient ingests the lethal dose. This is a somewhat bitter tasting slurry, and it must be swallowed completely and quickly – that is, within 30 seconds to two minutes from starting to ingest it. If the dose is taken slowly, the patient may fall asleep before ingesting an effective amount and death may not follow.

After ingesting the lethal drug, the patient may drink fruit juice or other liquid to offset the taste left by the drug. Most patients become unconscious in about 5 to 10 minutes after ingesting the drug, with a range from 1 to 60 minutes. They sleep peacefully until death ensues, with a median time of 25 to 30 minutes and a normal range of up to 3 hours after ingesting the drug. It may take longer (104 hours is the maximum reported), but once unconscious, patients sleep comfortably until they die.

Although some patients ingest the lethal dose alone or in a hospice, medically-assisted dying most often takes place in the home of the patient. Family members and friends are usually present at the time of ingestion to provide comfort and support to the patient.

Depending on the patient's wishes, the setting can be an opportunity to reflect on the good things in the life of a terminally ill patient and to exchange best wishes and good-byes with family members and those close to the patients. At the option of the patient, the setting may include the presence of the physician and a priest, and it may include prayers or religious rites. Such a gathering of family and friends can be an enriching celebration of the life of the patient as well as a time for final farewells.

There is no need to call 911 when the patient goes into a coma and subsequently dies. When a physician is not present, family members or friends can notify the patient's physician, the health-care facility, and a funeral home of the time of death.

When properly carried out, the cause of death by medically assisted dying is NOT recorded as suicide.[6] Instead, it is recorded on the patient's death certificate and on any official records as the underlying terminal illness for which the patient has been diagnosed or any other cause that has intervened, such as "respiratory failure" or "natural cause," such as that following a patient's removal from a ventilator.

For the terminally ill patients who died under Oregon's DWDA, 93.4 percent died at home, either their own home, their family's home, or the home of a friend; 4.9 percent died at a long-term care center or an assisted living or foster-care facility; 0.4 percent died in a hospital; and 1.3 percent died elsewhere.

Psychiatric studies of families and friends who had provided emotional and practical support for their loved ones' assisted deaths showed that participating in the process helped their bereavement. For some, their presence at the assisted death of a friend or family member was little more than an opportunity for bidding a fond farewell. For many, it was a celebration of a loved one's life, with retelling memories, reciting poems, and singing songs. Some who had initially opposed medically assisted dying changed their minds after witnessing the suffering their love ones had endured.[7]

Presence of Physician or Pharmacist at Death

In a medically assisted dying, neither the physician who prescribes a lethal dose of drugs nor the pharmacist who fills the prescription take any part in the terminally ill patient's act of freely and deliberately ingesting the lethal drug to end their life. They do not need to be present for a patient's ingesting the lethal prescription, though they may be present as guests if specifically invited by the patient.

Complications

The final act of ingesting the lethal drug has usually ended without complications. However, there have been difficulties in slightly less than one percent of the deaths. Patients who have not used an antiemetic medication beforehand have vomited some of the bitter-tasting drug, and their deaths have been delayed because of the reduced amount that remained. A few patients have interrupted ingesting the lethal dose and fallen asleep before ingesting enough to cause their deaths.

Medically Assisted Dying is a Choice

The participation of terminally ill patients, physicians, health providers (e.g., hospitals, hospices, nursing homes, hospices, or retirement communities), pharmacists, and witnesses in medically assisted dying is by the free and informed choice of each. No patient, physician, health provider, pharmacist, or witness that participates in the medically assisted dying of a terminally ill patient is compelled to do so. For example, if a physician does not wish to prescribe a dose of a lethal drug or a pharmacist does not wish to fill a prescription for a lethal drug, they have the legal right to refuse. In that case, the patient can choose a different physician who is willing to prescribe a lethal drug or a different pharmacist who is willing to fill the prescription.

A mentally competent and terminally ill adult is free to choose to participate in medically assisted dying. Neither doctors, nor pharmacists, nor the patients themselves are forced to participate in any step of medically assisted dying. Any one of them with moral objections may refuse to participate.

Hospitals have the legal right to allow its patients to choose a lethal drug to end their lives or not. They may also deny any physician who uses the hospital or its facilities to help a patient participate in any step of medically assisted dying, such as writing a prescription for a lethal drug. Most Catholic hospitals at the time of writing are opposed to medically assisted dying, and they do not allow it in their procedures or by a physician treating a patient in the hospital. *However, by law they are obliged to provide patients with information for alternate sources of drugs and for facilities that will provide the services they refuse to provide themselves.*

Using Lethal Medications to Continue Living

Not every terminally ill patient who receives the lethal drug will ingest it to end their process of dying. In applications of the law to date, only approximately two-thirds of eligible patients were in this category. For the other one-third, simply possessing the lethal drug restored enough autonomy over their bodies that they chose to continue their lives on their own terms. Many of these continued to live until they died from their terminal illness — most often within the six months of their diagnoses — or from other causes. A few lived for a couple of years after receiving the lethal drugs, despite the shorter life expectancy diagnosed. Several are reported to have lived until the age of 102.

As Philip Nitschke, an Australian physician and advocate for the right to die, once said, "[G]iving people access to a means of feeling that they're back in control of this issue is actually a way of prolonging life. It may seem paradoxical, but what we find is when people feel that they're back in control, they're less likely to do desperate things."[8]

The consequences of using medically assisted dying to obtain lethal doses of medication can be good whether or not terminally ill patients ingest the doses. For those who do ingest the lethal drug, it cuts short the pain and distress of dying. For those who do not, life continues, with pain and distress accepted so long as the lethal dose is available and restores a patient's dignity and personal autonomy. Thus, the consequences of medically assisted dying laws can be a rewarding and compassionate proposition for terminally ill patients and for their families and friends regardless of how they use the lethal drugs.

Non-Coverage for Neurodegenerative Diseases

Patients suffering from a neurodegenerative diseases (e.g.. Alzheimer's, Parkinson's, Huntington's, and amyotrophic lateral sclerosis) are not eligible to apply for medically assisted dying in the United States. This is because although such diseases are incurable, they are not fatal, and access to medically assisted dying requires a patient to be being terminally ill, with a prognosis of not more than six months to live because of a *fatal* disease or condition they have.

Roughly 10 million Americans have either Alzheimer's (5.7 million), Parkinson's (3.3 million), or other neurodegenerative diseases (1.0 million). They are the "untouchables" who have no recourse to medically assisted dying. Many fall victims of dementia, and eventually they die from other causes. They die *with* the degenerative disease, not *because* of it.

About 90 percent of Americans with a neurodegenerative disease are seniors, aged 65 years or older. Their life expectancy after the initial diagnosis of dementia is about 8 to 12 years. Those in the advanced stages of dementia have no personality, no memory, and no ability to speak for themselves; they are no more than living shells whose existence depends on some 15 to 20 million caregivers who provide unpaid assistance. They have no benefit to others except nursing home operators. They will eventually die of other causes than the neurodegenerative disease.

In the meantime, they take a heavy psychological toll on unprepared family members, especially on elderly spouses.

Many couples promise to help one another avoid such an ending, only to find themselves helpless when faced with its reality. As a result of the ineligibility of individuals with neurodegenerative diseases for medically assisted dying, there are countless sad stories of an elderly husband or wife spooning food into the mouth of an aged spouse with a neurodegenerative disease for month after month and year after year, helping them bathe or go to the toilet, and unable to converse with them because the other can no longer hear, think, or speak.

Caregivers suffer from depression as they watch the disease taking its toll on a loved one, and they become concerned about maintaining their own health. A typical story of a mercy killing that is played out over-and-over is the murder of a woman in her 60s or 70s with Alzheimer's disease whose husband, bereft by his wife's long-time illness, smothers her with a pillow. Such an ending is a result of not allowing people suffering from a neurodegenerative disease to end their suffering — and the agony of their family — by not legalizing medically assisted dying for patients with neurode-generative diseases.

Legal advocates are active in both Oregon and California to amend the laws for medically assisted dying to include coverage for individuals with neurodegenerative diseases.

SUICIDE

There are unfortunate misunderstandings about the definition of suicide that contribute to misunderstandings about medically assisted dying. The misuse of the term suicide, whether unintended or intentional, has led to much unwarranted opposition to medically assisted dying.

Definition of Suicide

Suicide is *not* simply taking one's own life. Suicide is more correctly defined as taking one's own life *intentionally* and *freely*, Note the words "intentionally" and "freely." They are very important for understanding why medically-assisted dying is *not* suicide. Whatever alternate name one chooses to use for a medically assisted dying law, it should not suggest or imply that it is or has anything to do with suicide.

"Intentionally," as used in the definition of suicide, means that the person committing the act of suicide fully intended that their act would result in their death — that the act was done intentionally, not accidentally, and not from a misunderstanding of the act's consequences. "Freely," as used in the definition, means that the person ending their own life was *not compelled* by a force beyond their control. (The word "deliberately" is sometimes used in place of "intentionally," and the word "voluntarily" is sometime used in place of "freely.")

Most states no longer classify suicide as a crime, since anyone who commits suicide is beyond the reach of the law. However, all states define aiding, assisting, or encouraging another individual to take their own life as a crime with potentially heavy penalties. (In a few states, suicide continues to be recognized as a crime by common law, and it may affect the rights of a beneficiary or claimant to the estate of the one who committed suicide, depending on whether they were of sound mind at the time.)

Suicide is generally stigmatized and discouraged. A few states make attempted suicide a crime. However, prosecution is rare, especially when the offender is terminally ill.

Why "Intentionally" and "Freely" are Important Words in the Definition of Suicide

The individuals who leaped from the high rooms of skyscrapers in New York City during the terrorist attack of September 11, 2001 did *not* commit suicide — even though they deliberately hurled themselves from great heights and knew that their death would follow instantly on hitting the pavement below.

What they intentionally did was a sane and reasonable alternative to enduring a slow, painful death by being burned alive by the fires in the rooms they leaped from. Their deaths were not caused by a choice they were free to make. Their intent was to escape a period of dying that was worse than jumping to their deaths, and they were compelled to make that choice by the agony they foresaw by burning to death. They were compelled to cause their deaths by the surrounding circumstances. Their deaths are therefore NOT recognized or recorded as suicides because their intent was NOT to kill themselves. Rather than choosing their actions freely, they did what they did under compulsion by circumstances from which they could not otherwise escape.

To put it simply, they preferred a quick, violent *death* to a slow and painful *dying*.

The reasons that competent terminally ill patients choose medically assisted dying to end their lives, such as the loss of autonomy over their lives, the inability to take part in activities that make life enjoyable, incontinence and the inability to control body functions, physical pain, or the fear of physical pain, are all recognized by the states that have legalized medically assisted dying as *substantive* reasons for seeking death *without* the stigma of suicide. Their death certificates properly list the cause of their death as their terminal illness or other intervening cause, *not* as suicide. That is, the existence of a compelling reason to end one's life can be a legally substantive *exception* to the act of taking one's own life in the meaning of suicide.

To repeat: When properly conducted according to the provisions of state law regulating it, medically assisted dying is *not* suicide. Nor is it homicide, murder or euthanasia. It is a means of escaping a tortured dying that is felt to be worse than death itself.

Misuse of the Term Suicide

The laws that have been enacted to legalize medically assisted dying are often misnamed "physician-assisted suicide" or some other term that includes the word "suicide." This misuse of the term "suicide" when speaking or writing of laws that have been enacted to make medically assisted dying legal are either due to ignorance or are attempts to discredit what is legal.

To repeat once more: Medically assisted dying is neither a form of suicide nor is it murder, homicide, or euthanasia. It is proper and legal in states where voters or legislators have enacted laws to legalize it and where patients, doctors and anyone else who participates in it follows rigid procedures to prevent abuses or misuse.

Suicide in the United States

Suicide is one of the leading causes of death in the United States. Table 1 shows the number and percentage distribution of suicides in 2015 for the total population and by sex and the method used. Corrected for population size, the annual number of suicides in the United States has increased from 10.5 per 100,000 population in 1999 to 13.0 in 2014, a significant increase of 24 percent over a period of only 14 years, as previously noted

Table 1: Suicides in the United States in 2015
(National Institute of Mental Health)

Method	Total Population		Male	Female
	Number	Percent	Percent	Percent
Firearm	22,018	49.8	55.6	33.4
Asphyxiation	11,855	26.8	10.0	30.5
Poisoning	6,816	15.4	26.9	26.7
Other	3,504	7.9	7.4	9.4
Total	44,193			

17

In 2015, a total of 44,193 Americans was reported as having died by suicide, and suicide was the tenth leading cause of death in the United States. Almost half (49.8%) of the suicides were by gunshot. The other principal methods were suffocation (26.8%) and poisoning (15.4%). The balance (7.9%) were by other means.

Many suicides are individuals who were depressed or were desperate to end the pain from terminal illnesses that could not be relieved by palliative care. Dying with dignity surrounded by family and friends is much better than an ugly suicide, which still carries a stigma with it.

For comparison, the number of deaths in 2015 from ingesting lethal medical doses under Death with Dignity type laws was less than 310 — that is, approximately 0.70 percent of the 44,193 who committed suicide in the United States the same year.

The number of fatalities in the United States during the year 2015 due to other causes were approximately as follows:

- Homicides (murder and manslaughter): 15,700
- Gun related (suicides and homicides): About 32,750
- Traffic and road accidents: 38,300 (Plus 4.4 million injured)
- Drug related: 52,504

Anyone truly concerned about the sanctity of life or the financial and emotional costs of end-of-life conditions for terminally ill patients, their families, and their friends can make better choices for spending their time or money to improve our society than opposing medically assisted dying laws. One might start, for example, by funding programs to provide psychological counseling for suicidal individuals that help avoid their committing suicide.

Suicide in the Past as a Crime against the State

Not many years ago, suicide was a crime against the state, and committing suicide could have very serious consequences. Even though a person who had committed suicide was beyond the reach of the law, there was a stigma attached to it, and there could still be nasty treatments of the corpse and the fate of the person's property or family members.

In ancient Athens, as related in the Wikipedia article about suicide legislation, "a person who had died by suicide (without the approval of the state) was denied the honors of a normal burial. The person would be buried alone, on the outskirts of the city, without a headstone or marker. A criminal ordinance issued by the French monarch Louis XIV in 1670 was far more severe in its punishment;

the dead person's body was drawn through the streets, face down, and then hung or thrown on a garbage heap. Additionally, all of the person's property was confiscated."[9]

Some monarchs and religious rulers of ancient Rome and medieval Japan treated suicide as a defiant act of extreme personal freedom against their "divine rights" as rulers. They used their power over their subjects for their own personal benefit rather than for their subjects' well-being, and they used religion to uphold their command as masters and superiors over their subjects. Until the late 20th century, suicide had a strong stigma attached to it and was considered a mark of shame or disgrace on a family's honor.

Today, none of the 50 states treat suicide as a crime against the state. It is, however, a common law crime in some states and, as mentioned earlier, it can have legal consequences. It can, for example, bar recovery for the late suicidal person's family in a lawsuit unless the suicidal person can be proven to have been of unsound mind.

Although suicide is no longer a crime, the act of aiding, assisting or encouraging another to take their own life *is* a crime.

Medially assisted dying has become a socially acceptable form of death, and suicide itself no longer carries a strong stigma of shame as it had in the past. For the most complete written discussion of suicide, see Derek Humphry's book *Final Exit: The Practicalities of Self-Deliverance and Assisted Suicide for the Dying,* a best-seller when first published in 1991 and now in its third edition (2010).

Voluntary Suicide by Refusing Food and Drink

U.S. citizens have the right to refuse life-support care needed for their survival. Also, if unwanted life-support care has been provided, they have the legal right to have it removed, even though its removal will lead to their death. For example, a competent terminally ill patient who is kept alive by artificial means (e.g., a breathing or feeding tube inserted into the person's body or an attachment to life-support equipment) has a constitutional right to have it removed and they be allowed to die.

This right to refuse medical intervention extends to refusing food and drink, even though doing so will cause the patient to die. This right is known as voluntarily stopping eating and drinking (VSED). It is a legitimate alternative to medically assisted dying and is legal throughout the United States. It is an accepted means of hastening death.[10]

The right to reject healthcare essential to keep a patient alive is well protected by court decisions at various levels, including the United States Supreme Court. In the case of *Cruzan v. Director, Missouri Department of Health* (1990), Justice Antonin Scalia of the United States Supreme Court pointed out in his concurrence with the majority opinion that making it legal for a patient to refuse medical treatment that was essential to keep them alive was equivalent to legalizing the right to commit suicide – which, he added, is. not a due process right protected by the Constitution. This raises the logical question: If patients have a constitutional right, guaranteed by the Fourteenth Amendment, to *refuse* unwanted medical care necessary to end their suffering, why are they not guaranteed a constitutional right to *use* medical care they want for the same purpose?

The court has held that the two situations are distinctly different in their intentions, and that an individual's right to refuse life support, even though their death will follow, does not imply a reciprocal right to use medical assistance to end one's suffering by causing their death. (The Cruzan case and another with like support are discussed in Chapter 4.)

While clinical physicians clearly have the legal right to discuss voluntarily stopping eating and drinking (VSED) with their patients and that patients have the legal right to request it, it is preferable that patients who feel they are ready to die should initiate the request to use it. Once the process begins, the patient remains lucid until falling into a coma after about two days. While still lucid, the patient can change their mind and stop the process. When done properly, VSED is an ethical, moral, and legal way for a patient to end their suffering or distress.

Voluntarily stopping eating and drinking has been available for decades. It is being used with increasing frequency to end the lives of individuals who are terminally ill or who have lost the will to live. It is an option in states that have not yet legalized medically assisted dying.

Compared to medically assisted dying, VSED has certain advantages:

- It is legal in all states.
- It is simpler. There is no mandatory waiting period to begin the process.
- It has fewer restrictions to its use.

- There is no need to find a physician who will prescribe a lethal drug nor a pharmacist who can and will provide it.
- There is no need to purchase an expensive lethal drug.

Once a person stops taking food or drink, they die of dehydration in one to two weeks. During this time, palliative care may continue to provide appropriate help, including control of symptoms and distress. Small amounts of water may be used for mouth comfort, to prevent lips from cracking, or to assist in swallowing pills. The person goes into a coma after two or three days without water or other fluid.

Although voluntarily stopping food and drink can be done at home without aid, it is best done in a clinic, nursing home, or hospice where clinical help and moral support are available. With proper care, voluntary suspension of eating and drinking need not lead to an agonizing and extended suffering.[11]

Death by dehydration is regarded by some as better than medically assisted dying with respect to personal integrity or asserting one's self-determination, or for its ready access (e.g., the delays with complying with the safeguards against abuse), or for the high cost of a dose of a lethal drug.

EUTHANASIA

Euthanasia is the direct termination of life by a physical act performed by a person upon another individual who requests help to relieve intractable or burdensome pain and suffering while dying. When done by a compassionate person, the action causing death is called "mercy killing." When a physician aids or assists an individual to terminate their life, it is called "euthanasia" or "physician-assisted suicide" in the strict, literal meaning of the latter name. (Be aware that the name "physician-assisted suicide" is often *misused* for what is correctly named "medically assisted dying.")

Euthanasia (or "physician-assisted suicide" in the strict, literal meaning of that term) is a crime in the United States. It is *not* legalized by the enactment of medically assisted dying laws, which do *not* allow a physician to administer a lethal dose directly unless specifically exempted by a court for a terminally ill patient who is unable to swallow.

The Netherlands is well known for euthanasia. The first known case of euthanasia there was in the early 1950s, when a physician performed euthanasia on his own brother. The brother was in the terminal stage of a disease that caused a great deal of severe

pain, and he repeatedly asked his brother for help to end his suffering. This was followed by other cases of euthanasia that drew the attention of the public and raised advocacy for its legalization.

In the 1980s, roughly three decades after the first case, the Netherlands codified a set of conditions that legalized what they called "termination of life on demand." The Netherlands law is the most liberal law that regulates euthanasia in Europe.[12] It permits euthanasia under the following conditions:

- The request originates from the patient and is given by him or her voluntarily and freely.
- The patient suffers intolerable pain, which cannot be alleviated by palliation or medical treatment.
- The patient is aware of their medical condition and has a good understanding of its perspective for their future.
- There is no other legal alternative to end the patient's suffering.
- The doctor who is to perform an act of euthanasia has consulted with a colleague who is both experienced in the field of end-of-life health care, has examined the patient, and agrees that all conditions are met for euthanasia,
- Euthanasia is performed with the necessary care.

Euthanasia in the Netherlands is subject to controls. A doctor carrying out euthanasia must fill out certain forms and submit them, with all required documents attached, to state or local authorities, such as a municipal pathologist. Unless doctors follow legal procedures and submit their required documentation, they may not be protected from prosecution for criminal action. On the surface, the intent of the legal caveats or controls imposed on the use of euthanasia in the Netherlands is much like the intent of the controls imposed on the use of medically assisted dying in the United States.[13]

Besides the Netherlands, medically assisted dying and euthanasia are now legal in Belgium, Colombia, Luxembourg, India, and Canada. Support for these end-of-life options is increasing in Western Europe and decreasing in central and Eastern Europe. Typical terminally ill patients are older, white, and well-educated, and more than 70 percent of the terminally ill patients are suffering from cancer.

SOME PAST HISTORY
AND A LOOK TO THE FUTURE

As discussed in Chapter 4, Dr. Jack Kevorkian's use of euthanasia in the 1980s and 1990s was a loud, well-publicized call for action to provide compassionate end-of-life care for terminally ill patients in the United States. Kevorkian's public advocacy of the right-to-die movement had been preceded by the formation of the Euthanasia Society of America in 1938. Its purpose was to foster the dissemination of information about the lawful termination of human life by painless means to avoid unnecessary suffering. It changed its name several times – to the Euthanasia Educational Council (1967), to Concern for Dying (1978), and to other names before ceasing operation in 2004 as the Partnership for Caring.

In 1980, the national right-to-die organization known as the Hemlock Society USA was founded by Derek Humphry. Humphrey's 1991 book *Final Exit* became a best-selling manual for committing suicide. The national membership of the Hemlock Society grew to 40,000 with eighty chapters. It changed its name to End of Life Choices in 2002. In 2003, End of Life Choices merged with the Compassion in Dying Federation and was renamed Compassion & Choices. Compassion & Choices has become the leading advocate for medically assisted dying in the United States.

A second organization, the Death with Dignity National Center (or Death with Dignity for short), was founded in 2004 to advocate for medically assisted dying. It is a collaboration of three political action groups that united in 1997 to enact Oregon's Death with Dignity Act of 1998 — the Oregon Death with Dignity Alliance, the Dignity Legal Defense and Education Center, and the Death with Dignity National Center.

While advocates and opponents of medically assisted dying continue their efforts, medical science continues to extend lifetimes. Studies of population genetics and evolutionary biology, and the role of genes and deoxyribonucleic acid (DNA) research on stem cell regeneration and DNA technologies have helped researchers understand and manipulate the genetic instructions and roles for the growth, development, functioning and reproduction of all known living organisms including humans. Studies of stem cells now allow researchers to control the regeneration of organs and tissue that have been damaged by illness or accidents, such as new skin tissue that can be grafted on to burn victims. We may soon find that life longevity has extended lives to 120 or 130 years. The consequences to our healthcare and financial pension systems are ominous and need to be addressed now.

CONCLUDING COMMENTS

In the last century, medical science has changed the scenario for the general populace from relatively short lives and quick deaths to long lives and prolonged dying.

The intent of a terminally ill patient who chooses medically assisted dying is not to die. It is rather to shorten a long and distressing period that can only end in death.

For most terminally ill patients, pain palliation and hospice care provide relatively peaceful and acceptable ends to their lives. For a significant number of others who face intense pain and suffering, particularly during the final period of dying, medically assisted dying offers an option for ending their dying process with dignity — under their own terms and at a time and in a setting of their own choice. Without access to medically assisted dying, the only acceptable alternative for thousands of them each year is suicide —that is, death by asphyxiation, a gunshot, poisoning, jumping from a tall structure, or voluntarily stopping to eat or drink, thereby dying by a slow process of dehydration or starving.

The consequence of medically assisted dying is *not* an ugly suicide. It typically ends in a celebration, with family members and close friends gathered together, embracing one another in a compassionate and edifying expression of love and the beauty of life. Medically assisted dying is a much better alternative for everyone than suicide.

Life should be good. When old age, illness, or accidents change it from good to bad — so painful or stressful that it is no longer worth living — medically assisted dying provides a compassionate and dignified ending.

# # # # #

Chapter 2

EXPERIENCE OF STATES WITH
MEDICALLY ASSISTED DYING LAWS

On November 8, 1994, voters in Oregon passed the state's Death with Dignity Act (DWDA) to make Oregon the first state in the United States — and one of the earliest in the world — to legalize medically assisted dying (MAD). However, because of attempts to repeal DWDA, its implementation was delayed until early 1998, slightly more than three years after its enactment.

Oregon's Death with Dignity Act allows adult residents who are terminally ill to end their lives through the self-administration of lethal medications prescribed by physicians. The patients ingest the lethal drugs at a time and under the conditions of their choice, which is most often in their homes in the presence of their families and close friends.

Since the passage and implementation of Oregon's Death with Dignity Act, five more states have enacted similar laws, either by voter initiatives (Washington, 2008; California, 2015; Colorado, 2016; and Hawaii, 2018), or by enactment by a state legislature (Vermont, 2013). In addition, the right for residents to use medically assisted dying has been upheld by court decision (Montana, 2009). In addition, the district of Washington, D.C. has also enacted a medically assisted dying law by voter initiative (2017). Initiatives are also being pursued in other states at the time of writing.

Table 2 shows the main results to the time of writing in states with medically assisted dying laws. It shows the dates on which implementation of the laws began. Data is given for the total number of terminally ill patients who received lethal drugs and the number and percentage of those who ingested the drugs and died, The data is complete from the dates of implementing the laws to the end of 2018 for Oregon and to the end of 2017 for the other states.

The public health departments of the various states with medically assisted dying laws issue annual reports with extensive compilations of the statistics associated with the implementation of the laws. Short summaries of some of these are given in this chapter. For full details, the annual reports of the state public health departments can be downloaded from their web sites.

Table 2 – Main Results for Medically Assisted Dying Laws

Jurisdiction	Method for Enacting	Implemen-tation Date	Total Number of Lethal Doses Issued	Total Number of Lethal Doses Ingested	Percent Ingested
Oregon	Voters	11/4/1997	2,216	1,459	65.8
Washington	Voters	3/5/2009	1,387	1,006	72.5
Vermont	Legist.	5/20/2013	52	29	55.8
California	Voters	6/9/2016	768	487	63.4
Colorado	Voters	12/16/2016	197	n.a.	--
Dist. Columbia	Voters	6/6/2017	0	0	--
Hawaii	Voters	1/1/2019	0	0	--
		Totals	4,620	2,981 *	67.4 *

* Does not include "ingested" result for Colorado
Data for Oregon and Colorado includes 2018. Others end with 2017.

This chapter also recounts some experiences of the states for passing laws to legalize medically assisted dying. It discusses the opposition that voters and their representatives had to overcome in passing, defending, and implementing the laws. It includes details in several instances to illustrate the attempts and maneuverings of politicians, legislatures, and others with special interests to thwart the wishes of voters — even in states where independent polls had shown that large majorities of voters were in favor of medically assisted dying laws.

This chapter thus celebrates the triumphs and victories of politically active citizens who persevered over intimidation and obstacles to enact progressive legislation for our social and political system of democracy. The fulfilment of their work lies with the terminally ill patients who died with dignity rather than by ending their lives in pain and despair, so deep that others with similar end-of-life conditions have been driven to ugly suicides.

For comparison, a final short section discusses Canada's legalization and nationwide implementation of a similar law, which it names medical aid in dying (MAID).

OREGON

Oregon's Measure 16, titled the "Death with Dignity Act," (DWDA), was a voters' initiative to legalize medically assisted dying. It sets forth the legal framework within which a competent terminally-ill adult can request a prescription for medication for the purpose of ending their life in a humane and dignified manner. Measure 16 was passed in a general election on November 8, 1994, when voters approved it with 627,980 votes (51.3 percent) in favor and 596,018 votes (48.7 percent) against.

Measure 16 was meant to be implemented the following month. However, it proved to be one of the most controversial ballot measures in Oregon's history, and it was not implemented until October 27, 1997.

Initial Measure and Injunction to Block Its Implementation

On November 23, 1994, two weeks after the enactment of Measure 16 for Oregon's Death with Dignity Act and before it was placed into effect, a class action suit was filed in the Federal Court of the Ninth District to ban the law. The suit was filed by supporters of the National Right to Life Committee[1] on the grounds that Measure 16 violated their equal protection and due process rights under the Fourteenth Amendment of the United States Constitution, their free exercise of religion and freedom of association rights under the First Amendment, and their statutory rights under the Americans with Disabilities Act of 1990.

On December 7, 1994, Judge Michael R. Hogan of the federal court for the Ninth District placed a temporary restraining order on Measure 16. In the meantime, the group that had organized the voter initiative for the enactment of Oregon's law formed Oregon's Death with Dignity Legal Defense and Education Center, the forerunner of the Death with Dignity National Center. On December 12, this group filed a motion in support of Measure 16. Judge Hogan of the federal court responded by extending the restraining order and then, on December 27, 1994, issued a temporary injunction against the implementation of the Measure.[2]

Throughout 1995, Oregon's Death with Dignity Act moved back and forth in the Ninth Circuit Court of Appeals on behalf of Michael Vernon, a terminally ill patient. On August 3, Judge Hogan ruled Measure 16 was unconstitutional and made the injunction against its implementation permanent. Essentially, the district court found "that the Act violated the Equal Protection Clause because it provided insufficient safeguards to prevent against an incompetent or depressed terminally-ill adult from committing suicide, thereby irrationally depriving terminally-ill adults of safeguards against suicide provided to adults who are not terminally ill."[3]

On November 24, 1995, Oregon's Death with Dignity group filed a brief with the Circuit Court of Appeals appealing Judge

Hogan's granting a permanent injunction against implementing Measure 16.

On March 7, 1996, Oregon's Death with Dignity requested a stay of the injunction against Measure 16. The Ninth District Court of Appeals denied the request and sent the question back to Judge Hogan, who again denied the motion to stay the injunction against Measure 16. This denial was appealed.

On February 27, 1997, the United States Court of Appeals, Ninth Circuit concluded that "the federal courts do not have jurisdiction … over Plaintiffs' claims. Accordingly, we vacate the judgment of the district court and remand with instructions to dismiss Plaintiffs' complaint for lack of jurisdiction."[4]

In the meantime, legislators for the state of Oregon were taking action to repeal Measure 16. On January 28-29, 1997, the Family Law Subcommittee of Oregon's House of Representatives held informational meetings on Measure 16. On February 17, the Oregon State Legislature introduced seven bills to repeal, refer to committee, delay, or alter Measure 16, the state's Death with Dignity Act.

Later in 1997, Oregon's Legislative Assembly voted to submit Measure 51, which would have repealed Measure 16, to a special election. Opponents to Measure 51 pointed out that because voters had already passed Measure 16, asking them to change their minds and vote against it in favor of its repeal was disrespectful.

At a special election on November 4, 1997, Oregon voters rejected Measure 51, thereby reinstating Measure 16, the state's Death with Dignity Act. The vote was 666,275 (59.9%) against Measure 51 and only 445,830 (40.1%) in favor. This was a significant increase in the percentage of voters in favor of DWDA when Measure 16 was first approved three years earlier. Implementation followed shortly thereafter.

During 1998, the first full year of implementation of Oregon's DWDA, 24 terminally ill residents of Oregon received prescriptions for lethal doses. Of these, sixteen ingested the doses and ended the process of dying with their dignity intact. The law continued in effect for the next six years, with annual increases in the number of participants each year.

A Second Attempt to Block Oregon's DWDA

In the meantime, former Missouri Senator John Ashcroft was confirmed on February 2, 2001 as President George W. Bush's appointee to succeed Janet Reno as U.S. Attorney General. Ashcroft alleged that medically assisted dying was not a legitimate purpose for prescribing legal drugs and vowed to prosecute physicians who he claimed were violating federal law.

On November 6, 2001, Ashcroft tried to block Oregon's law by issuing his "Ashcroft Directive," which authorized Drug Enforcing Agents (DEA) to investigate and prosecute doctors who prescribed federally controlled drugs to help terminally ill patients end their lives. Two days later, U.S. District Judge Robert Jones issued an injunction against the U.S. Attorney General's order until arguments were heard. On April 17, 2002, Judge Jones ruled that the U.S. Justice Department lacked the authority to overturn an Oregon law that allowed physicians to participate in the state's DWDA.

On September 23, 2002, barely five months later, Attorney General Ashcroft filed an appeal in *Oregon v. Ashcroft* with the 9th U.S. Circuit Court of Appeals to suspend a physician's license for prescribing life-ending medications covered in the Controlled Substances Act (CSA). On May 7, 2003, oral arguments were heard in the Court of Appeals, and on May 26, 2004, a three-judge panel asserted: "We hold that the Ashcroft Directive is unlawful and non-enforceable because it violates the plain language of the CSA, contravenes Congress' express legislative intent, and oversteps the bounds of the Attorney General's statutory authority."[5]

On July 12, 2004, Attorney General John Ashcroft appealed the ruling and requested an 11-member panel to rehear the case of *Oregon v. Ashcroft*. On August 11, the Circuit Court rejected Ashcroft's request. On November 9, 2004, the deadline for an appeal, Ashcroft filed his petition with the U. S. Supreme Court, and later that day he announced his retirement from the Department of Justice. He was succeeded as Attorney General by Alberto Gonzales. (After resigning as Attorney General, Ashcroft founded the Ashcroft Group, a Washington D. C. lobbying firm.)

Late in 2004, a federal court ruled that when Congress passed the Controlled Substance Act, it did not authorize the Attorney General to penalize physicians who followed state laws in prescribing federally regulated drugs. The appeals court held that the federal law on drug control was intended to halt drug traffickers, not to regulate physicians or the practice of medicine. (Historically, the licensing of physicians and regulating medical care have been left to the individual states rather than the federal government.)

In February 2005, the U.S. Supreme Court granted the Department of Justice's request for a hearing of *Gonzales v. Oregon,* No. 04-623 (formerly *Oregon v. Ashcroft,* with Ashcroft's name replaced by Gonzalez, who had replaced him as Attorney General). Oral arguments were heard on October 5, 2005. In a split decision on January 17, 2006, the Supreme Court voted 6-3 to uphold Oregon's DWDA for medically assisted dying. It ruled that former Attorney General John Ashcroft, acting on behalf of the Bush administration, had overstepped his authority in seeking to punish doctors who had prescribed drugs to help terminally ill patients end their dying.

In its decision, the Supreme Court of the United States held that the state law of Oregon supersedes federal authority to regulate physicians. Chief Justice John Roberts and Associate Justices Anthony Scalia and Clarence Thomas dissented. An article in the Washington Times quoted Senator Ron Wyden (D-OR) as saying the Supreme Court's ruling was "a significant victory" that stops the Bush administration's efforts to "wrest control of decisions rightfully left to the states and individuals."[6]

Before, between, and after these two successes in court, there was a continuing battle and several setbacks in implementing Oregon's Death with Dignity Act. Claims were tossed about *without convincing evidence* that the law had a "slippery slope" that would lead to wrong or unacceptable results for certain groups or individuals, such as disabled persons, the elderly, the poor, and heirs seeking to profit from a patient's estate. In fact, the medically assisted dying laws of Oregon and other states have an array of caveats to protect against such abuses or misuse, and there are no substantiated cases of harm caused by such laws.

Thus, an independent study reported in the *Journal of Medical Ethics* for October 2007 *found no evidence* that Oregon's Death with Dignity Act had "heightened [the] risk for the elderly, women, the uninsured, ... people with low educational status, the poor, the physically disabled or chronically ill, minors, people with psychiatric illnesses, including depression, or racial or ethnic minorities, compared with background populations. The only group with heightened risk was people with AIDS."[7]

No attacks against Oregon's Death with Dignity Act have proved valid, and it has become the model for medically assisted dying laws in several other states. It is also the basis for the documentary film "How to Die" in Oregon, which was released in January 2011 at the 27th Sundance Film Festival, where it won the Grand Jury Prize for Documentaries. The film began airing on Home Box Office (HBO) later that year.

The Brittany Maynard Story

The best-known individual of those who moved to Oregon to avail themselves of the state's medically assisted dying law is Brittany Lauren Maynard (1984-2014),[8] a Californian with late- stage terminal brain tumor. She was only 29 years old when she ended her life by ingesting a lethal prescription in Oregon on November 1, 2014. Her story was told in newspapers and television programs nationwide, and it was instrumental in publicizing the end-of-life difficulties faced by young people as well as older ones.

Maynard earned a bachelor's degree in psychology from the University of California in Berkeley in 2006 and a master's degree in education from the University of California in Irvine in 2010. She taught at orphanages in Nepal, and she traveled widely in Vietnam, Cambodia, and other parts of Southeast Asia. She married Daniel ("Dan") Estaban Diaz in September 2012, and the two planned to have a family.

In January 2014, Maynard was diagnosed with grade 2 astrocytoma, a type of brain cancer that usually does not spread outside the brain and spinal cord. After a partial craniotomy and resection of her temporal lobe, the cancer returned. In April 2014, her diagnosis was changed to glioblastoma or grade 4 astrocytoma, and she was given a prognosis of six months to live.

Maynard and her husband created the Brittany Maynard Fund and partnered with the organization Compassion & Choices to advocate for legislation for medically assisted dying. Because California did not yet have such a law, Maynard and her family moved to Oregon to take advantage of that state's Death with Dignity Law. She would have preferred to die with her family at home in California.

In the weeks preceding her death, Maynard became the face of the campaign led by Compassion & Choices to enact medically assisted laws in the United States. At a time when the average person seeking medically assisted dying in Oregon was around 71 years of age, Maynard was a young, vivacious, and attractive 29. In her final posting to Facebook, she wrote: "Today is the day I have chosen to pass away with dignity in the face of my terminal illness, the terrible brain cancer that has taken so much from me … but would have taken so much more. … Goodbye world. Spread cheer. Pay it forward!"[9]

Successful Operation of Oregon's Death with Dignity Act

Each year, Oregon's Public Health Division prepares an annual report that includes statistical information on the operation of the state's Death with Dignity Act. Figure 1 summarizes the activity during 2018. A total of 249 terminally ill patients received prescriptions for a lethal drug during the year. Of these, 158 patients plus another 11 who had received lethal doses in the prior year ingested the lethal doses. Of these 169 patients, 168 patients died from ingesting the lethal drugs, and one patient regained consciousness and died later of their underlying illness.

48 patients who received lethal doses in 2018 did not ingest them and die. Instead, they continued to live, with some measure of their autonomy restored by possession of the lethal drug.

Final results were not complete for another 43 patients who received lethal doses in 2018. Fourteen of these had died, but it is not known if the cause of their deaths was due to ingesting the lethal drugs or to other causes. For the remaining 29 deaths, the ingestion status is pending.

Table 3 shows a set of consolidated statistics from the 21 years from 1998, the first full year of the law's implementation, to the end of 2018. During these twenty-one years, a total of 2,217 terminally ill patients in Oregon received lethal medications. Of these, 1,459 patients (65.8 percent, or roughly two-thirds of the total) ended their lives by ingesting the lethal prescriptions.

For comparison, the 1,459 terminally ill patients who ingested the lethal drugs and died with dignity over the 21-year period were slightly less than 0.038 percent of Oregon's population of 3.352 million in 1998, the first year of the state's implementation of its DWD Act. The stampede of out-of-state patients to Oregon to take advantage of the state's DWD Act that was predicted by foes of medically assisted dying has simply not materialized. In fact, Oregon's DWD Act has been used sparingly — hardly noticeable compared to the most common causes of death.

The other 758 terminally ill patients (34.2 percent of the total who received lethal drugs) had enough of their autonomy restored that they chose to continue their lives with their dignity intact until they died from their diagnosed terminal illnesses or other causes. A few continued to live for two years or more after receiving prescriptions for lethal drugs.[10,11]

Figure 1 –Operation of Oregon's Law in 2018
(Oregon Department of Health)

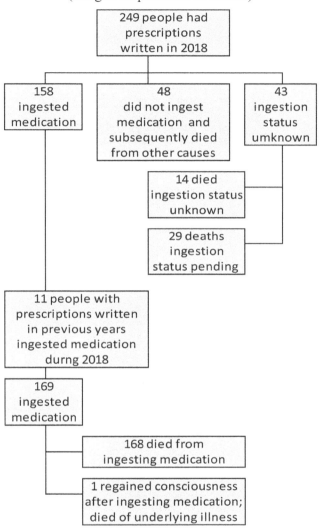

249 people had prescriptions written in 2018

158 ingested medication

48 did not ingest medication and subsequently died from other causes

43 ingestion status umknown

14 died ingestion status unknown

29 deaths ingestion status pending

11 people with prescriptions written in previous years ingested medication durng 2018

169 ingested medication

168 died from ingesting medication

1 regained consciousness after ingesting medication; died of underlying illness

While the general trend shown in Table 3 is a year-to-year increase in the number of terminally ill patients who receive lethal doses, the percentage of recipients who ingest the doses to end their dying scatters randomly about an average of 65.3 percent (or roughly two-thirds). The other roughly one-third of the recipients of lethal drugs do not ingest them but continue their lives until their deaths, usually from their terminal illnesses and within or shortly beyond their six months diagnosis to live. Why exactly they changed their minds and chose not to use the lethal doses is not known.

Table 3: Number of Recipients of Lethal Doses
and How They Used Their Doses
(Oregon State Department of Health)

Year	Received Doses, Number	Used the Lethal Doses They Received			
		To Die		To Live	
		Number	Percent	Number	Percent
1998	24	16	66.7%	8	33.3%
1999	33	27	81.8%	6	18.2%
2000	39	27	69.2%	12	30.8%
2001	44	21	47.7%	23	52.3%
2002	58	38	65.5%	20	34.5%
2003	68	42	61.8%	26	38.2%
2004	60	37	61.7%	23	38.3%
2005	65	38	58.5%	27	41.5%
2006	65	46	70.8%	19	29.2%
2007	85	49	57.6%	36	42.4%
2008	88	60	68.2%	28	31.8%
2009	95	59	62.1%	36	37.9%
2010	97	65	67.0%	32	33.0%
2011	114	71	62.3%	43	37.7%
2012	116	85	73.3%	31	26.7%
2013	121	73	60.3%	48	39.7%
2014	155	105	67.7%	50	32.3%
2015	218	135	61.9%	83	38.1%
2016	204	139	68.1%	65	31.9%
2017	219	158	72.1%	61	27.9%
2018	249	168	67.5%	81	32.5%
Total	2217	1459	65.8%	758	34.2%
		Average	65.3%		34.7%
		Median	66.7%		33.3%
		Minimum	47.7%		18.2%
		Maximum	81.8%		52.3%

The Bumpy Road of Implementation

Figure 2 plots the data in Table 3 to examine the general trend of the number of terminally ill patients who received lethal drugs each year from 1998 to 2016 to increase with time.

Rather than a single trend line, the data points in Figure 2 show four distinctly different periods with times and conditions as follows:

• Period 1 (1998-2003): Implementation of Oregon's DWDA began in 1998, and the number of terminally ill patients who received lethal prescriptions each year increased at an average rate of 7.5 per year for the next five years.

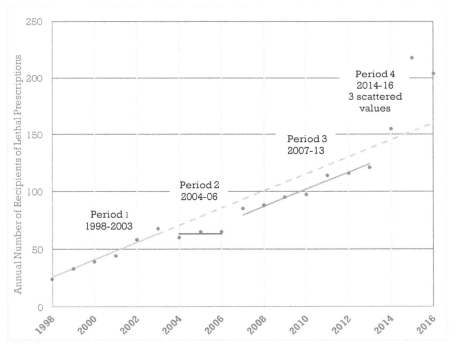

Figure 2 – Number of Recipients Receiving Lethal Doses
in Oregon each Year from 1998 to 2016

• Period 2 (2004-2007): During this period, the number of terminally ill patients who received lethal doses leveled off at around 65 per year. This change from the previous period was due to Attorney General John Ashcroft's unsuccessful attempt to scuttle the law by restricting the use of lethal drugs reserved under the Controlled Substance Act to the federal government,

- Period 3 (2008-2013): With the Supreme Court's ruling against Attorney General Ashcroft, the year-to-year increase in the number of lethal doses dispensed to terminally ill Oregon residents returned to the earlier average rate of 7.5 per year, with an offset or drop of 13.5 persons per year below the earlier trend line. (That is, the drop of the solid trend line during period 3 from the dashed projection of the earlier line was due to the disruption and uncertainty caused by Ashcroft's opposition – what one might term the "Ashcroft penalty," so to speak).
- Period 4 (2014-2017): The sudden and irregular increases from 2013 to 2014 (a year-to-year jump of 34 patients receiving lethal drugs) and from 2014 to 2015 (a jump of 63 patients) were due to the publicity surrounding the death of Brittany Maynard under Oregon's law on November 1, 2014. The high point of 218 patients' receiving doses was reached in 2015 and was followed by a drop to 204 patients in 2016. This was followed by a rise of 14 to a total of 218 patients in 2017 (as indicated by the data in Table 2).

Many terminally ill patients of the time, and many more of the future, are indebted to Brittany Maynard for her example in facing her final days of life and ending her suffering on her own terms, with dauntless courage and dignity — a lesson for all of us.

Reasons for Choosing to Receive Lethal Doses

Table 4 summarizes the reasons why terminally ill patients chose to obtain doses of lethal drugs to end their lives under Oregon's DWDA.

The data for Table 4 was generated from questionnaires on which patients who had received doses of drugs were asked why they chose to use medically assisted dying as an end-of-life option. The responders checked off as many of the reasons on the list that applied to them. At the top of the responses were the loss of autonomy and the inability to engage in activities that made life enjoyable or worth living, including concern that these might increase in the future. The term "autonomy" literally means, "living by one's own laws" (from autos "self" + nomos "law"). It can be defined as the ability of a person to make their own decisions and to live and enjoy life on their own terms. These two reasons were checked by approximately 95 percent of the patients who received lethal doses.

Table 4: Reasons for Terminally Ill Oregon Residents'
Ingesting Lethal Medications to End Dying
(Oregon State Department of Health)

Year(s)	2018		1998-2018	
Deaths from Ingesting Lethal Medication	168		1,459	
End of Life Concerns	N	Pct	N	Pct
Loss of autonomy	154	95.1	1,322	95.5
Less able to engage in an enjoyable life	152	95.6	1,300	94.6
Loss of dignity	112	79.4	989	87.4
Loss of control over body functions	62	46.3	647	56.5
Burden on family, friends, or caregivers	91	63.6	654	51.9
Inadequate pain control or concerns for it	43	31.2	375	29.8
Financial implications of treatment	9	7.3	57	4.7

For comparison, physical pain was checked by around 30 percent of the respondents. Concern for pain was mainly for future pain, which can become agonizing for the later stages of some forms of cancer, rather than immediate pain at the time of entering a medically assisted dying program. Since a patient is terminally ill and facing death, immediate pain is less a concern.

The preponderance of concern for autonomy factors rather than pain was confirmed by a study at the Oregon Health & Science University. One patient, on being asked the most important thing for them in their dying days, responded "I want to do it on my terms. I want to choose the place and time. I want my friends to be there. And I don't want to linger and dwindle and rot in front of myself."[12]

The percentages for "Loss of dignity" and "Loss of control over body functions" have both been lower for 2018, whereas the percentage for "Burden on family, friends, or caregivers" has increased. Pain has much less importance for choosing to end one's life, probably because palliation methods to reduce pain have been so successful. Financial implications are of relatively little concern.

Table 5 summarizes the terminal illnesses of patients who received lethal doses. The data shows that some form of cancer is the primary terminal illness of patients who seek medically assisted dying. According to the testimony presented in one of the legal cases: "Cancer usually progresses steadily and slowly. The cancer patient is fully aware of his or her present suffering and anticipates certain future suffering. The terminal cancer patient faces a future that can be terrifying. Near the end, the cancer patient is usually bedridden, rapidly losing mental and physical functions, often in excruciating, unrelenting pain. Pain management at this stage often requires the patient to choose between enduring unrelenting pain or surrendering an alert mental state because the dose of drugs adequate to alleviate the pain will impair consciousness. Many patients will choose one or the other of these options; however, some patients do not want to end their days either racked with pain or in a drug-induced stupor. For some patients pain cannot be managed even with aggressive use of drugs."[13]

Table 5: Underlying Illnesses of Terminally Ill Patients
Who Died after Ingesting Lethal Drugs (1998-2018)
(Oregon State Department of Health)

Cancer	Percent
Lip, oral cavity, and pharynx	2.1%
Digestive organs	19.9%
Pancreas	6.9%
Colon	5.9%
Other digestive organs	7.2%
Lung and bronchus	16.0%
Breast	7.0%
Female genital organs	5.8%
Prostate	4.3%
Urinary tract	2.9%
Eye, brain, and central nervous system	3.2%
Lymphoma and leukemia	4.5%
Other types of cancer	16.1%
Total Cancer	**75.9%**
Neurological disease	11.0%
Respiratory disease	5.1%
Heart or circulatory disease	4.5%
Infectious disease (e.g. HIV/AIDS)	0.9%
Other illnesses	2.6%
Total illnesses other than cancer	**24.1%**
Total	**100.0%**

Table 6 identifies the characteristics of patients who received doses of lethal drugs to end their lives under Oregon's Death with Dignity Law during the 21 years between January 1, 1998 and December 31, 2018. By and large, the typical patient was white, was either married or had been married and was divorced or widowed, was well educated, had been under hospice care, and died at home.

Table 6: Characteristics of Patients Who Received Lethal Doses
(Oregon State Department of Health)

- **Sex**: 52.3% male, 47.7% Female
- **Age**: Ranged from as young as 25 years to as old as 102 years, with a median of 72 years and 8.3% younger than 55 years of age
- **Race**: 96.4% of patients were white, 1.4% were Asian, 1.0% were Hispanic, and remaining 1.2% were others.
- **Marital Status**: 46.1% were married (including registered domestic partner), 22.0% were widowed, 24.1% were divorced, and 7.9% had never married.
- **Education**: 42.8% had a college baccalaureate degree or higher, 9.0% had an associate degree, 21.2% had some college education, 22.0% had graduated from high school, and 5.0% had less than a high-school education.
- **Place of Death**: 92.4% of patients died at home — either their own home, their family's home, or the home of a friend; 5.0% died at a long-term care center or an assisted living or foster-care facility; 1.0% died in a nursing home, 0.3% died in a hospital, 0.1% died in a hospice, and 1.3% died elsewhere.
- **Hospice Care**: 90.2% were enrolled in hospice care, and the other 9.8% were not.

How Patients Used their Doses of Lethal Drugs

As discussed earlier, about two-thirds of those who received lethal drugs used them to end their lives. For this group, the time from the first request for a lethal dose to its ingestion varied, with a median time of 48 days (approximately 7 weeks or nearly two months). This means that most patients who received lethal drugs were in no hurry to use them, and the doses of lethal drugs were requested for future rather than immediate use. Their ingestion was put off until a patient's condition had deteriorated to such a loss of autonomy or other distress that a breaking point was reached and patients decided to end their suffering by dying.

While two-thirds of the terminally ill patients used their doses to end their lives of suffering, the other one-third of patients used their lethal doses to continue their lives, despite their suffering. The latter group did not ingest their lethal drugs, but simply possessing them restored enough of their immediate autonomy and control over their bodies so that they chose to continue to live. Most of this one-third died within six months or slightly longer of the causes for which they had been diagnosed as terminally ill. Some died between six months and a year after receiving the lethal drugs. A few continued to live for more than two years after receiving (but not ingesting) the lethal doses. Several terminally ill patients who had obtained lethal drugs continued to live until their deaths at the age of 102.

It is inspiring to this writer that such a relatively large fraction — about one-third of those who received lethal drugs — chose to continue to live. Despite their loss of enjoyment in life and any aches and pains or other distresses that had prompted them to consider ending their lives, restoring their sense of autonomy restored their wish to live.

Complications

Complications have been uncommon during the years that Oregon's DWDA has been in effect. Seven patients woke up after ingesting the lethal dose. Six of them later died of their diagnosed terminal illnesses, and one was still alive the following year. One patient, a very heavily set woman with a bowel blockage, failed to consume all the lethal dose in one or two minutes before falling asleep and stayed in a coma for 104 hours (slightly more than four days) before she passed away without waking up.

Swallowing anti-nausea medication before ingesting the lethal dose reduces the likelihood of gagging, having difficulty swallowing the lethal dose, or vomiting after swallowing it.

Participation by Physicians

Oregon has around 14,000 licensed physicians, and fewer than 1 percent of them have written lethal prescriptions under the state's Death with Dignity Act. Some physicians do not want to participate, and some are forbidden by the healthcare facilities that employ them, such as Catholic hospitals and companies whose leaders are opposed because of their strong religious beliefs.

WASHINGTON STATE

On November 4, 2008, voters in the state of Washington passed a Death with Dignity Act (Initiative 1000, codified as RCW 70.245) by a 57.8 percent to 42.2 percent margin, thereby making Washington the second state in the U.S. to allow terminally ill residents to end their lives by ingesting lethal doses of medication. The Washington DWDA is patterned after Oregon's, and it became effective on March 5, 2009. (A similar initiative had been rejected by Washington voters by a margin of 54 percent to 46 percent in 1991.)

Table 7 shows the growth in participation in Washington's DWDA — from 63 terminally ill residents of the state in 2000, the Act's first year of implementation, to 239 during 2016. As in Oregon, the general trend in Washington has been a year-to-year increase in the number of patients who used the law to obtain lethal doses, except for 2017, when 212 terminally ill patients did so.

Table 7: Annual Participation in Washington's
Death with Dignity Act
(Washington State Department of Health)

Year	Obtained Lethal Dose	Died from Ingesting Lethal Dose	
	Number	Number	Percent
2009	63	35	55.6%
2010	87	51	58.6%
2011	103	70	68.0%
2012	121	83	68.6%
2013	173	119	68.8%
2014	176	126	71.6%
2015	213	166	77.9%
2016	239	192	80.3%
2017	212	164	77.4%
Total	1387	1006	
		Average	72.5%

For comparison, the population of the state of Washington (est. 7,530,552 for 2018) is about 1.79 times that for Oregon (4,199,563).

Unlike Oregon, in all but 2017, the last year of data for Washington, both the *number* who received legal doses and the *percentage* of those who ingested the doses to end their dying process increased each year, and the percentage is higher than in Oregon,

Washington collected data on the reason for participating in the state's DWDA for only the first three years. The most common reason was the loss of autonomy, which was given by 100 percent of the participants in 2009 and dropped to 87 percent in 2011. Next was the loss of enjoyment in life (which varied between a high of 97

41

percent to a low of 87 percent), followed by a loss of dignity (which varied between 82 percent and 64 percent).

The youngest participant in Washington's DWDA was 20 years old, and the oldest was 101.

The Back-and-Forth Court Decisions and Appeals

The enactment of Washington's Death with Dignity Act followed a long battle in the courts that began in 1994, when a group of plaintiffs challenged the Washington state law (identified as RCW 9 A 36.060) that prohibited physician-assisted suicide, as medically assisted dying was then improperly named. The group of plaintiffs included three terminally ill patients, five physicians who treated them, and an organization named Compassion in Dying. This group asserted that Washington state's ban was unconstitutional on the grounds that it deprived mentally competent, terminally ill adults with no chance of recovery of a "liberty interest" that was constitutionally protected under the Fourteenth Amendment to the U.S. Constitution. This "liberty interest" gave them "the right to commit physician-assisted suicide [i.e. medically assisted dying] without undue governmental interference." The case was tried in the U.S. District Court for the Western District of Washington. On May 3, 1994, the U.S. District Court ruled in favor of the plaintiffs.[14]

In reaching its decision for the plaintiffs, the Washington District court noted that the United States Supreme Court had established through a long line of cases that personal decisions relating to marriage, procreation, contraception, family relationships, child rearing and education are matters involving the most intimate and personal choices a person may make in a lifetime. Such choices are central to personal dignity and autonomy, and they are central to the liberties protected by the Fourteenth Amendment. The court also noted that some of these, such as abortion and contraception, may offend the most basic principles of morality of many persons as individuals. However, the court's obligation is to define the liberty of all, not to mandate its own moral code.[15]

In expressing its decision, the Washington District Court declared RCW 9 A 36.060 unconstitutional because it "places an undue burden on the exercise of a protected Fourteenth Amendment liberty interest by terminally ill, mentally competent adults acting knowingly and voluntarily, without undue influence from third parties, who wish to commit physician-assisted suicide. The court further declares RCW 9 A. 36.060 unconstitutional because it violates the right to equal protection under the Fourteenth Amendment by prohibiting physician-assisted suicide (*i.e., medically assisted suicide*) while permitting the refusal or withdrawal of life support systems for terminally ill individuals."[16]

An appeal was filed with the United States Court of Appeals for the Ninth District, and on March 9, 1995, a two-judge panel of the Appeals Court reversed the decision of the Washington State District Court and reinstated the ban on medically assisted dying as constitutional.

However, on May 28, 1996, after rehearing the case *en banc* — that is, by the full court — the U.S. Court of Appeals for the Ninth Circuit reversed the earlier decision of the two-judge panel and affirmed the District Court's decision that declared RCW 9 A 36.060 unconstitutional and removed its prohibition of medically assisted dying.

In removing the ban on medically assisted dying enacted by the Washington legislature, the U.S. Court of Appeals "took into consideration the interests of the state in protecting life, preventing suicides, preventing undue, arbitrary, or unfair influences on an individual's decision to end his life, and ensuring the integrity of the medical profession. These interests were balanced against an individual's strong liberty interest in determining how and when one's life should end. The court recognized this interest after assessing the growing public support for assisted suicide [*i.e., medically assisted dying*], changes in the causes of death and medical advances, and Supreme Court cases addressing due process liberty interests. The court then determined that the state's interest, which could be protected by adopting sufficient safeguards, did not outweigh the severe burden placed on the terminally ill, and thus the statute as applied was unconstitutional."[17]

Finally, the Attorney General for Washington state petitioned the Supreme Court of the United States for a writ of *certiorari* — that is, for the U.S. Supreme Court to review the evidence, findings and decision of the Washington Ninth Circuit Appellate Court. The Supreme Court agreed to do so, and on January 8, 1997 it decided that the Due Process Clause of the Fourteenth Amendment did not include the right to commit assisted suicide — that is, medically assisted dying is not a fundamental "liberty interest"[18] guaranteed by the Fourteenth Amendment of the U.S. Constitution, and a terminally ill patient does not have a constitutional right to use medically assisted dying to end their suffering.

Chief Justice Rehnquist wrote the court's majority opinion, which reversed the decision of the Ninth Circuit Court that the ban on physician-assisted suicide (i.e., medically assisted dying) was a violation of the Due Process Clause of the Fourteenth Amendment. Instead, the U.S. Supreme Court upheld the law enacted by the Washington state legislature to ban or prohibit medically assisted dying (i.e., physician-assisted suicide).

The Supreme Court decision ended the merry-go-round of the series of court battles in which the repeal of the state law forbidding medically assisted dying was followed by a successful appeal to reinstate the ban, another appeal to repeal the law, another successful counter appeal, another successful appeal to repeal, finally ending in 1997 with the reinstatement of the state law to ban or prohibit medically assigned dying.

The series of court hearings continually used the incorrect and biased tern "physician-assisted suicide," which is a name for euthanasia, which is in fact illegal. This continues to create much misunderstanding and bias against what is properly termed "medically-assisted dying" or "medical aid in dying," which is a legal act in those states or jurisdictions that have passed legislation to make them legal, and it is NOT suicide.

The Supreme Court's decision was followed by a voter initiative that finally resulted in the enactment of Washington state's Death with Dignity act of 2008. That marked the end of a long back-and-forth battle in state and federal courts that was marked by a series of appeals and reversals. The final settlement by the United States Supreme Court, which recognized the rights of states in the matter, reinstated the ban or prohibition of medically assisted dying enacted by the state legislature. However, if their state legislators were opposed to medically assisted dying and would not enact a law that made medically assisted dying available to them, the voters of Washington state could enact one themselves — which is what they did following the Supreme Court's decision.

MONTANA

In 2009, in the case of *Baxter, et al. v. Montana, et al.*, the Montana Supreme Court, citing the state's Rights of the Terminally Ill Act, ruled that physicians may assist patients to end their lives by prescribing lethal medications for self-administration by the patients.

That is, Montana's existing law already gave physicians immunity from prosecution if they provided or withheld life-sustaining support as requested by terminally ill patients. Although the court's ruling does not specifically address medically assisted dying, it does confirm that it is legal.[19]

A case was brought before the Montana Supreme Court to determine whether or not the state's constitution guarantees that terminally ill patients have the right to obtain a prescription for a lethal drug to end their lives. The lead plaintiff in the case was Robert Baxter, a 75-year-old retired truck driver with lymphocytic leukemia, a terminal form of cancer. Baxter suffered from anemia, chronic fatigue, nausea, night sweats, infections, massively swollen glands, serious digestive problems, and pain. He had been treated with multiple rounds of chemotherapy, which typically become less effective as time passes. Baxter wanted the right to demand a prescription for a lethal drug to end his life when his suffering became unbearable.

Other named plaintiffs were board certified physicians who frequently treated terminally ill patients, and a national non-profit group, Compassion & Choices. The plaintiffs sued the state of Montana to declare the homicide statutes a denial of their constitutional right for medically assisted dying. In effect, they asked the Court to decide that the patient had a constitutional right to medically assisted dying.

The court sidestepped this issue and instead ruled on narrower grounds that neither legal precedent nor the state's statutes made such assistance illegal as being against public policy. In effect, the Court's ruling affirmed that it is legal for physicians to prescribe lethal doses to end the lives of their terminally ill patients.

Judge Dorothy McCarter of the Montana Supreme Court, in supporting the court's decision, opined that although "the Constitution confers no right to aid in ending one's life, … [the] constitutional rights of individual privacy and human dignity, taken together, encompass the right of a competent terminally-ill patient to die with dignity."[20]

Plaintiff Robert Baxter died on December 31, 2009, the same day the trial court issued its opinion — and, sadly, too late to benefit from the court's decision.

Subsequent to the decision of *Baxter v. Montana*, groups in Montana opposed to medically assisted dying have been trying to get the state legislature to overturn the court's decision by enacting a statute to ban it. At the same time, other groups that supported medically assisted dying are trying to get either voters or the state legislature to pass a law that codifies detailed provisions for medically assisted dying in the form of the Death with Dignity laws in Oregon and five other states besides Montana.

In 2015, in the absence of a statute that codified the procedure for medically assisted dying, the *Journal of Palliative Medicine* published a text titled "Clinical Criteria for Physician Aid in Dying" to guide physicians in Montana and other states without codified procedures.[21]

State legislators opposed to medically assisted dying have tried again and again to overturn the court's ruling. The fifth and latest attempt is bill HB 284. As of February 6, 2019, the bill was in the state's Judiciary Committee for hearing. If passed by the Montana State Legislature, the bill would criminalize medically assisted dying in Montana.

VERMONT

In May 2013, four months after its introduction in the Vermont Senate, the state's Act 39, titled "Patient Choice and Control at End of Life" was passed by both houses of the state's legislature and was signed by Governor Peter Shumlin. Vermont thus became the first state to legalize medically assisted dying through action by the state legislature rather than voter initiative (as in Oregon and Washington) or by court decision (as in Montana). Vermont's law went into effect immediately on the governor's signature.

The Act's passage was the culmination of a 10-year campaign by individuals organized as Patient Choices Vermont in collaboration with the national Death with Dignity organization (which, like Compassion & Choices, advocates for medically assisted dying laws). Like the medically assisted dying laws in Oregon and Washington, Vermont's law defines the directions that must be followed to provide strong safeguards against abuse.[22,23]

Following the law's passage, the Vermont Department of Health issued a "Patient's Bill of Rights" that listed all the options and choices physicians must inform their patients about relevant to their medical treatment. It also directed physicians to answer all of their patients' questions fully so that their patients could make fully informed decisions about the care they were to receive. The legality of this provision of Vermont's law was challenged in July 2016, by the Vermont Alliance for Ethical Healthcare and the Christian Medical and Dental Association, a Tennessee-based Christian healthcare group. Their suit claimed that the law infringed on a physician's freedom of speech on the grounds that it might oppose a physician's religious and ethical beliefs about the sanctity of human life.

In April 2017, Judge Geoffrey Crawford of the U.S. District Court dismissed the challenge and held that "physicians must inform patients of all choices and options relevant to their medical treatment."24

In May 2015, the Sunset Provision (Senate Bill 108, Act 27) on certain patient safeguards was removed.

As of June 30, 2017, 49 Vermont residents had received prescriptions for lethal drugs under the state's medically assisted dying law, and 29 of these (59.2%) had ingested the drugs to end their process of dying.

Later Legislative Action and Challenges

The opposition continued. Four bills were introduced in 2017 in Vermont's House of Representatives to restrict or modify the law passed four years earlier.

- HR 254 would require a physician to have a minimum of six months of experience with a patient before being allowed to prescribe a lethal drug rather than leaving it to the physician to decide if he or she has sufficient knowledge to make that decision. (This sort of opposition emphasizes the need for patients to plan ahead and document their end-of-life wishes and discuss issues with their families or friends while they are still competent.)
- HR 255 would require an independent witness to be present when a patient ingested the lethal drug.
- HR 298 would require a physician to consult with the Adult Protection Services Program before writing a prescription for a lethal drug and to document certain steps taken during the consultation.
- HR 320 would specify that physicians are not obliged to inform patients about their options under Vermont's medically assisted dying law (Act 39). On December 18, 2017, Judge Geoffrey W. Crawford of the U.S. District Court upheld Vermont's law by ruling that it is a physician's duty to provide full information about their end-of-life healthcare options and alternatives to terminally ill patients applying for a lethal drug to end their lives under Vermont's Act 39, *regardless of a physician's personal beliefs and opposition to doing so.*

CALIFORNIA

On June 9, 2016, California's End of Life Options Act (EOLOA) legalizing medically assisted dying became effective. Like Oregon's Death with Dignity Act of 1998, after which it is patterned, California's End of Life Options Act allows competent terminally ill adult patients of California to obtain lethal medication to end their suffering. Governor Jerry Brown, a Catholic, signed the Act into law on October 5, 2015,25 but opposition delayed its implementation until June 9, 2016. It has survived persistent opposition to overturn it based on a procedural change in enacting the law.

The Rocky Road to Legalization

California's End of Life Options Act was introduced in January 2015 by Senators Lois Wolk and Bill Monning as Senate Bill 128 after earlier attempts by voter initiatives and legislation had failed. After passage by the California Senate, the bill was held up in the Health Committee of the House of Representatives by intense and well-organized opposition led by the Roman Catholic diocese of Los Angeles. Although the American Medical Association also continued its opposition, many physicians and the California Medical Association, which represents physicians in the state, withdrew its opposition of long standing.

After the sponsors of the Senate Bill recognized their bill would fail if brought to a vote in the Health Committee of the House of Representatives, the bill was modified and reintroduced into a special committee on Health which Governor Jerry Brown had formed earlier. California's End of Life Options Act passed there, and it was then introduced for vote by the full House of Representatives. The House added its approval to the Senate's by a solid majority of 56.5 percent to 43.5 percent, and Governor Brown signed the Act into law on October 5, 2015.

Because the Bill had been approved by a special committee on Health rather than the House's regular Health Committee, the law's implementation was delayed until 90 days after the special committee's closing of all its assigned business. California's End of Life Options Act finally became effective and was implemented on June 9, 2016.

During the nearly 19 months from the law's initial implementation to December 31, 2017, 835 terminally ill patients received lethal drugs. Of these, 485 individuals (or 58.1 percent of the total) had ingested the lethal drugs as of December 31, 2017. This is a lower percentage rate of ingestion by those who received lethal drugs than the roughly 66.7 percent (or two thirds) in other states with medically assisted dying laws.

Opposition to California's End of Life Options Act

On June 8, 2016, the day before California's End of Life Option Act (EOLOA) took effect, two organizations — the American Academy of Medical Ethics and the Life Legal Defense Foundation — and six physicians filed a lawsuit against the Office of the District Attorney of Riverside County, California in the Superior Court of Riverside County to ban the law's implementation. The plaintiffs claimed that (1) the law violated the due process and equal protection guarantees of the United States' and California's constitutions because it failed to make rational distinctions between terminally ill adults and the majority of Californians who were not covered by the Act, and (2) the California legislature did not have the legal authority to pass the law during a special session on healthcare. The court rejected the plaintiffs' motions for a temporary restraining order and preliminary injunction, and the law went into effect.[26]

On June 16, 2017, slightly more than a year from the implementation of California's End of Life Options Act, a California Superior Court ruled that the lawsuit to overturn the Act would proceed to trial to determine the merits of the case. The trial on the lawsuit was long delayed.

On May 18, 2018, while the lawsuit awaited trial, the judge of the Superior Court in Riverside County, California issued a formal judgment that California's End of Life Options Act was unconstitutional because of the procedural technicality cited in the earlier case. He granted a five-day stay before the law would become ineffective, and the state's attorney general promptly filed an appeal. On May 25, 2018, the judge declared the law was no longer in effect. An appeal was filed with California's Fourth District Court of Appeals in Riverside County on June 1, and the court placed the law back into effect on June 15 while it awaited a hearing of the case.

On August 31, 2018, the Riverside County Superior Court of Appeals ruled tentatively on part one of the suit brought two years earlier, holding that the plaintiffs in that suit had no standing to bring the case and it should never have been allowed to proceed. It pointed out that the plaintiffs could not possibly speak for terminally ill patients who wished to avail themselves of medically assisted dying, even if they claimed to be doing so for the patients' benefit. If patients did not wish to use medically assisted dying, they were free not to request it. No one was forcing them to choose what California's End of Life Options Act made available to them.

A hearing on the tentative ruling of the Riverside County Superior Court of Appeal was held on October 8, 2018. On November 27, 2018, the Fourth Appellate District of California ruled against the plaintiff physicians in the case of *Ahn v. Hestrin* on the grounds that, since the physicians were both free to opt out of participating in the state's End-of-Life Options Act, the plaintiff physicians did not have legal standing to file their lawsuit challenging the Act and seeking to overturn it. However, the plaintiffs have the option of amending their suit and appealing the lower court's decision to the California Supreme Court. In the meantime, the Act remains in effect and doctors can write prescriptions for terminally ill patients' obtaining lethal drugs to end their suffering.

The legal fight was not over at the time of writing (February 21, 2019). The court might amend their tentative ruling, and it must still hear oral arguments and rule on the second issue — that the law was unconstitutional because of the manner in which it was passed. Ultimately, the plaintiffs could take appeal their claim to the California Supreme Court.

Meanwhile, on February 16, 2018, Senator Mike Morrell introduced Senate Bill 1336 in the California Legislature, another example of opposition. The Bill was a substantial amendment to the 2016 End of Life Options Act, and ostensibly it was meant to provide information needed to improve the understanding of end-of-life issues in California. Opponents contended that the Bill's requirements added unnecessary steps that would have made it all but impossible for terminally ill patients to use medically assisted dying. Senate Bill 1336 was defeated at a committee hearing.

Statistical Results for 2016 and 2017

From June 8 to December 31 of 2016, 258 terminally ill patients started the end-of-life options act, of which 67 patients dropped out in favor of hospice, pain palliation, or other healthcare. Figure 3 summarizes what happened to the other 191 patients who obtained prescriptions for lethal drugs.

In 2017, the following year, 632 terminally ill patients started the end-of-life options act, of which 55 patients dropped out in favor of hospice, pain palliation, or other healthcare. That left 577 terminally ill patients who had prescriptions for lethal drugs written for them.

Figure 3 – End-of-Life Options Results
for First Seven Months of 2016

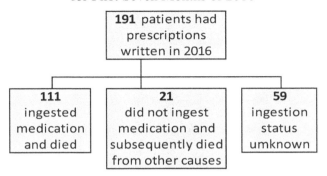

Figure 4 summarizes what happened to the other 577 patients who obtained prescriptions for lethal drugs and certain patients from 2016.

Figure 4 – End-of-Life Options Results for 2017

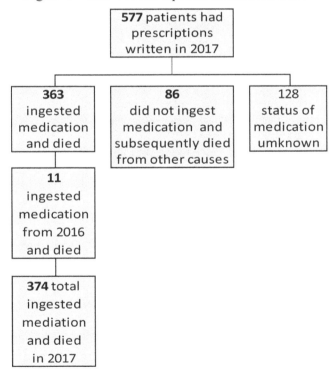

Of the 577 terminally ill patients who obtained lethal drugs to end their suffering during 2017,[27] 363 ingested their lethal doses in 2017 and died. In addition, 11 patients who had received lethal doses in 2016 also ingested their does in 2017 and died. This gives a total of 374 patients who died in 2017 from using the state's End-of-Life Options Act.

Another 86 patients from the 577 that had received lethal drugs in 2017 did not ingest the lethal drugs and died from their terminal illnesses or other causes. The status of the remaining patients and their medications had not been determined as of the date of the report.

Table 8 presents data on the characteristics of terminally ill patients who received doses of lethal drugs in the period from June 8, 2016 to December 31, 2017.

Table 8 – Characteristics of Terminally Ill Patients of California Who Received Medically Assisted Dying Action in 2017

- **Sex**: 47.1% male, 50.8% female, 21% unknown.
- **Age**: 9.6% under 60 years, 48.4% from 60 to 79 years, and 42.0% over 80 years. Median age was 74 years.
- **Race or Ethnicity**: 88.9% of patients were white, 5.1% were Asian, Native American or Pacific Islander, 3.9% were Hispanic, 0.0% were African-American, and 2.1% were unknown.
- **Marital Status**: 45.5% were married (including registered domestic partner), 23.0 % were widowed, 23.8% were divorced, and 7.7% had never married.
- **Education**: 57.2% had a college baccalaureate degree or higher, 17.9% had some college education but no degree, 21.4% had high school or general education development, and 3.5% had no high-school diploma.
- **End-of-Life Care**: 83.4% were enrolled in hospice and/or palliative care, 11.2% were not enrolled, and 5.4% were unknown.

COLORADO

Two attempts to pass a medically assisted dying act by legislative action by the Colorado House of Representatives failed, the first in 2015 (HB 15-1135) and the second in January 2016 (HB 16-1054). A bill identical to the latter was also introduced in the Colorado Senate in January 2016 (SB 16-025), but it also failed in February.

On November 8, 2016, Colorado voters took over and passed Proposition 106, the "End of Life Options Act," by a margin of 65 to 35 percent (almost a 2-to-1 margin). The law went into effect of December 16, 2016. According to a survey made two months before the voters voted, 70 percent of Coloradans supported the proposed law, with 46 percent strongly favoring it.

The following year, opponents of the new voter-enacted law introduced a new bill in the Colorado legislature to amend the law by requiring that either the attending physician or hospice medical director sign the death certificate of a terminally ill patient who had ended their life by ingesting a prescribed lethal dose. That bill died in committee.

During 2017, the first year of operation of Colorado's End-of-Life Options Act, 72 terminally ill patients received lethal prescriptions for aid-in-dying. During the second year, 2018, this number rose to 125 terminally ill patients, a 74 percent increase.

Colorado does not follow up to identify the patients who ingest their lethal prescriptions and those who do not.

WASHINGTON, D.C.

On January 15, 2015, the "Death with Dignity Act of 2015" was introduced into the Council of the District of Columbia. It was modeled on Oregon's law and polls showed that 67 percent of the district's population favored it. The bill passed its final reading on November 15, 2016 by a margin of 11 to 2. On December 19, 2016, the Mayor of Washington, D.C. signed the bill, and on January 6, 2017, the bill was passed on to the U.S. Congress for a required 30-day review and approval.

On January 12, 2017, Republican representatives in both the House and Senate introduced resolutions that disapproved D.C.'s law. However, because neither resolution reached the House or Senate floors for discussion and action by the February 17 deadline, D.C.'s law became effective the following day. The Act's implementation was scheduled to start on June 6, 2017. However, later in June, the D.C. Department of Health advised D.C. residents waiting to begin the steps to obtain a lethal dose that healthcare providers were unprepared to implement the Act's provisions.

On July 13, 2017, the Appropriations Committee of the House of Representatives of the U.S. Congress voted to repeal the act and to bar any funding to implement the District's program. The vote was 28-to-24, split along party lines in favor of the Republicans.

Threats of repealing the District of Columbia's Death with Dignity Act have caused doctors, pharmacists, and other members of D.C.'s healthcare system to hesitate before investing their time to develop policies and procedures for participating in the Act's implementation, which might fail. Thus, the future of D.C.'s Death with Dignity Act was uncertain at the time of writing. Meanwhile, the painful lives of terminally ill patients in our nation's capital continue in a state of uncertainty that only adds to their misery.[28]

HAWAII

Hawaii's "Our Care, Our Choice Act" passed both Houses of Hawaii's Legislature with huge margins: 39-to-12 (76.5%) in the House of Representatives and 23-to-2 (92.0%) in the Senate. On April 5, 2018, Hawaii Governor David Ige signed the Act into law and Hawaii became the seventh U.S. state, along with the District of Columbia, to have a Death with Dignity statute. The law will go into effect on January 1, 2019.

CANADA

This section provides information for medically assisted dying in Canada for comparison to similar laws in the United States.

On June 5, 2014, about sixteen years after the implementation of the state of Oregon's Death with Dignity Act, the Province of Quebec became the first Canadian province to legalize medically assisted dying. The law passed in the National Assembly by a solid majority of 94 to 22 votes. The strong majority vote in favor of prompted the Canadian Parliament and Supreme Court to work together to enact a legal basis for medically assisted dying for the entire nation of Canada.

They began with Section 7 of the Canadian Charter of Rights and Freedoms, which provides that "everyone has the right to life, liberty and security of the person and the right not to be deprived thereof except in accordance with the principles of fundamental justice."[29] On February 6, 2016 in a unanimous decision in the case of Carter v. Canada, the Supreme Court declared that the sections of the nation's Criminal Code that prohibited assistance in terminating life by means of medical assistance in dying (MAID) "infringe upon the right to life, liberty and security of the person for individuals who want access to MAID."[30] The court declared that those section of the Charter "are void insofar as they prohibit physician-assisted death for a competent adult person who (1) clearly consents to the termination of life, and (2) has a grievous and irremediable medical conditions (including an illness, disease, or disability) that causes enduring suffering that is intolerable to the individual in the circumstances of his or her condition."[31]

On April 16, 2016, in its response to the Supreme Court decision, the Canadian Parliament amended its Criminal Code to establish exemptions for physicians, nurse practitioners, pharma-cists and certain others in the implementation of the nation's medical assistance in dying (MAID) law. The Canadian law gives to any Canadian for whom a natural death is "reasonably foreseeable" or "incurable" the right to medically assisted dying. Patients are eligible if they have been verified by two physicians to comply with the following conditions:

- are competent adults – that is, are at least 18 years of age, and are mentally capable of making decisions and giving assent;
- have a serious illness, disease or disability;
- are in an advanced state of decline that cannot be reversed;
- are experiencing unbearable physical or mental suffering from their illness, disease, disability or state of decline that cannot be relieved by means or conditions the patient considers acceptable;
- and, considering all of their medical conditions and circumstances, their natural death has become reasonably foreseeable.

Note that Canada does not require a prognosis for the specific length of time remaining — only that death is reasonably foreseeable.

Canadian law also allows two types of medical assistance, each of which must include either a physician or nurse practitioner who:

- provides or prescribes a drug that the eligible person takes themselves, in order to bring about their own death. This option is known as self-administered medical assistance in dying. (It was previously incorrectly termed medically assisted suicide, physician aided suicide, or assisted suicide.; or,
- directly administers a substance that causes the patient's death, such as an injection of a drug. This option is known as clinician-administered medical assistance in dying. (It was previously known as voluntary euthanasia and had been illegal.)

The Canadian law became effective January 1, l016. followed by a 6-month delay give hospitals and physicians time to meet administrative requirements and to set up clinical protocols. Implementation of the law began on June 17, 2016.

Three reports for the preceding six-month periods have been issued to date. Table 9 indicates the number of individuals who availed themselves of the law from June 17, 2016 to December 31, 2017, the last period for which statistics were available.[32]

Table 9 – Deaths during First Three 6-Month Periods

Period	Date	Number	Increase
1st	June 17 to December 31, 2016	875	
2nd	Jan. 1 to June 30, 2017	1,086	24.1%
3rd	July 1 to December 31, 2017	1,525	26.8%
	Total	3,486	

As in the United States, cancer was by far the most frequent medical conditions for which medical aid in dying was chosen in Canada, accounting for approximately 65 percent of all cases. This was followed by respiratory or circulatory conditions (16 percent) and neurodegenerative diseases (10 percent).

The settings in which assisted dying took place varied between 40 to 42 percent for hospitals, 40 to 43 percent for patients' homes, and the balance in long-term care facilities or nursing homes.

CONCLUDING COMMENTS

At the time of publication of this book, medically assisted dying had completed 21 years of successful operation in the state of Oregon and, to lesser times, in seven other jurisdictions. During that time, more than four thousand residents of United States received lethal drugs to end suffering at the ends of their lives. Close to two-thirds of those residents ingested the drugs and died, most at home in the company of family and friends. The other one-third continued to live with their autonomy restored until their terminal illnesses or some other cause finally terminated it. The bereavement periods for the families and friends were lessened in both duration and intensity by their participation in the compassionate and dignified deaths of their loved ones.

The record of successes has been achieved without the abuses feared by opponents of medically assisted dying. In the more than 40 years of combined experience in seven states and the District of Columbia to the end of 2017, there have been no authenticated reports of abuse or coercion.

Not only have medically assisted dying laws been successes for patients and their loved ones, they have had a broader benefit to the entire system of healthcare. For example, in the words of one physician with 45 years of experience in family care, they have "catalyzed improvement in end-of-life care, a much broader discussion of end-of-life care issues, more frequent conversations between physicians and patients about their end-of-life care wishes and goals, doctor-patient relationships, and the awareness of and participation in hospice and palliative care services."[33]

Yet, despite the successes the laws have had, and despite the fact that a significant majority of Americans favor medically assisted dying — in fact, public polls shows the percentage of Americans in favor is around 70 percent — only six more states and the District of Columbia have enacted similar laws in the twenty years since Oregon enacted its Death with Dignity law, the first and the model for similar laws that followed.

Voter apathy is one factor. For example, the percentage of the American electorate who voted in the 2016 presidential election was about 58 percent of eligible voters, nearly the same as for the presidential election four years earlier. To put it another way, more than 4 out of 10 eligible voters did not vote in a presidential election.

Medically assisted dying has also been successful in Canada, where its implementation began in the province of Quebec in 2016, sixteen years after it began in the United States in the state of Oregon. It quickly spread across the entire nation of Canada. Two factors that stand out in comparing the acceptance of medically assisted dying in the two nations are: (1) its quick acceptance in the province of Quebec, where Catholics are a majority of the population, and (2) its quick spread across the entire nation of Canada.

Political and religious opposition to medically assisted dying laws has been much stronger in the United States than in Canada and across much of Europe. Despite the wishes of most residents, there is strong opposition against medically assisted dying by misguided individuals, religious prelates, and conservative senators and representatives in state legislatures.

Medically assisted dying has been a change from the past. It is a change brought about by the dedicated work of voters and legislators who fought for it — and will continue the fight until it is legal nationwide.

The opposition to making that change is discussed in the next chapter.

# # # # #

Chapter 3

OPPOSITION TO
MEDICALLY ASSISTED DYING

"To change" can be the most difficult verb in the entire dictionary for a person to do.

In this chapter, the opponents to change are the politicians and churchmen opposed to legalizing medically assisted dying because of their political views or religious beliefs. They often use language to create a bias against change. For example, they use nasty-sounding names that can trigger opposition, such as "physician-assisted suicide," for what is properly described as "medically assisted dying" or "medical aid in dying."

The name "physician-assisted suicide" caused much opposition by physicians and their professional societies. It suggested a role that was entirely opposite to what physicians had dedicated themselves. Fortunately, the deception is now understood for what it was, and the majority of physicians are now in favor of medically assisted dying,

This chapter might be viewed as a retrospective of the preceding chapter — in the sense that it is a celebration of victory for those political activists who worked hard, over a period of years, to overcome opposition to change for the better. They persevered in preparing voter initiatives or in persuading state legislators to prepare bills that were voted into the enactment of laws for medically assisted dying in their states of residence. All honor to them.

POLITICAL OPPOSITION

Opponents of medically assisted dying laws claim that the laws lack sufficient safeguards to protect terminally-ill patients who might be abused because they are elderly, disabled, incompetent, poor, or members of an ethnic minority. These claims are not aimed directly at the substance of the laws, which is to legalize medically assisted dying as an end-of-life option. They express legitimate concerns that each state must manage, administer, and control their laws so as to avoid abuses or misuse. For example, many elderly patients who are diagnosed as terminally ill have poor decision-making abilities.[2] Rather than being allowed to choose medically assisted dying, they should be treated for depression or provided with some other alternative such as hospice care and pain palliation. Such alternate care is actually being provided as part of the routine of medically assisted dying laws. [1,2]

The fact is that the seven states with medically assisted dying have now accumulated a total of 46 years of experience and have yet to experience their first adjudicated failure to operate improperly. The procedures to avoid "the slippery" have proven adequate. They are discussed in the following sections, in which a properly appointed surrogate may function in place of a patient if the patient is not competent.

Depressed or Mentally Incompetent Patients

The procedure for obtaining a lethal drug to end their suffering begins when a patient who has been diagnosed as terminally ill and likely to die of an incurable illness in less than six months makes an oral request for medically assisted dying. The request might be made to the patient's primary care physician, for example, or to a nurse or other staff member of a nursing home that is taking care of the patient, or to a staff member of a hospital or its emergency room where the patient has been taken. The oral request for medically assisted dying is followed by a terminally ill patient's meeting with a physician (designated the attending physician), who is usually the patient's primary care physician and has some prior experience with the patient.

The first step is for the attending physician to determine the patient's condition – that is, the patient is terminally ill and is not expected to live more than six months, and the patient is neither depressed nor mentally incompetent. If a patient satisfies these conditions, they are referred to a second or consulting physician who repeats the examination.

If either the attending or consulting physician feels the patient might be depressed, suicidal. or mentally incompetent, the patient is referred to a psychiatrist or licensed psychologist to evaluate the patient's condition and competence to choose medically assisted dying and their freedom from depression. If the psychiatrist or psychologist believes the patient may be mentally depressed or incompetent, the patient is referred to a mental care facility for relief of depression or for mental care. Otherwise, if the patient is evaluated as mentally competent and free of depression or suicidal tendencies, the process continues to the next step.

If the patient is judged during the foregoing to have the combination of knowledge, temperament, emotional stability, and logical skills to assess the conditions of their dying and the consequences of choosing medically assisted dying, the attending and consulting physician discuss alternatives that the patient might consider. The alternatives include hospice care at home or in a hospice or nursing home, where the care may include psychiatric counseling, pain palliation, or pain sedation. Many terminally ill patients change their minds at this point and choose an alternative to medically assisted dying. If they persist in choosing medially assisted dying, the procedure continues.

Not less than fifteen calendar days after both physicians have determined a terminally ill patient is mentally competent to choose medically assisted dying, the patient makes a second oral request for medically assisted dying. The attending and consulting physicians then meet separately a second time with the patient and discuss the alternatives again. If the patient continues to choose medically assisted dying, the patient must sign a written request to do so. The patient's signature must be signed by the attending physician and by two witnesses, one of which must not be a relative of the patient or have any interest in the patient's estate or be a member of a hospice or nursing facility which has been caring for the patient.

After all steps have been completed, the attending physician must wait 48 hours to allow for any change of the patient's mind before writing a prescription for a lethal drug for the patient. The patient can then acquire a lethal drug and ingest it later at a time and in a setting of their choice, or the patient can retain the lethal prescription and continue to live until they die of their terminal illness or other cause.

The procedure for a terminally ill patient's acquiring a lethal drug can take a month or two from the patient's initial decision to do so. Some patients have died during this period.

Six-Month Prognosis for Death

It's estimated that three quarters of Americans will die from serious debilitating illnesses that can take 2 to 5 years to result in death. Many will die in much shorter times from the time they have been judged terminally ill, and some will take 10 years, and a few even longer.

For example, some forms of cancer periodically go into remission, during which the signs and symptoms of their cancer are reduced. Others are kept alive by periodic radiation and chemotherapy and, by such means, they may stay alive for five years or more. The final stage may then be short — perhaps a few days or weeks — before death is judged to be imminent.

A final period of acute pain or agony is probably the biggest worry of cancer patients, who comprise about 70% of patients enrolled in medically assisted dying. For them, a short prognosis to live is favorable, because they can complete the process for obtaining a lethal drug in the event their cancer should suddenly worsen and impose an agonizing period of pain before death. Once they have a lethal drug, they can delay ingesting it as long as they wish, secure in the autonomy it gives them for ending their suffering at a time and under conditions of their own choice.

Critics of medically assisted dying point out that physicians are unable to forecast their patients remaining lifetimes accurately, even though they may have been attending their patients for many years. Doctors themselves admit their inability to forecast deaths accurately. Most often they err on the side of longer forecasts than what actually happens, probably so as not to upset patients with shorter forecasts. All too often, an ailing patient with a long-term prognosis will suddenly take a turn for the worse and die in a few days or a week or two — too late to begin and complete the procedure for obtaining a lethal drug under the legal requirements of medically assisted dying laws.

No single criterion, such as a prognosis of death in not more than six months, can possibly be proper for everyone. If an error is to be made, *it should be made in favor of the best interests of the patients* – that is, as short a prognosis for death as appears possible or reasonably foreseeable in order to have enough time to obtain a lethal drug for ingestion.

Patients are the ones who suffer the most from prognoses that are too long, which means that they will endure pains and distress longer than proper before being allowed to receive lethal doses to end their suffering. An unfortunate scenario that has often played out is a patient who has been diagnosed as terminally ill and has applied for medically assisted dying but dies before they can complete the process for obtaining a lethal drug to end their suffering.

Typically, it takes more than a month or two between a successful patient's taking the first step to request a lethal drug under a state's medically assisted dying law and receive the drug. There is a further delay in arranging a time with family and friends present when the patient ingests the drug and dies. Many patients have died of their terminal illness before receiving the lethal drug or, having received it, before they have completed arrangements for a final meeting with family and friends and ingesting it.

Inadequate End-of-Life Counseling

Critics contend that some attending physicians are poorly prepared to discuss the deeply personal, end-of-life wants and needs of terminally ill patients and to help them choose the end-of-life option that is best for them. Others feel physicians do not take enough time to do this well, especially for patients who are elderly, disabled, or a minority, and to discuss the full range of options available for handling them so they can make good decisions. The alternatives include, for example; pain palliation; palliation sedation; hospice care at the patient's home, nursing home, or hospice; voluntarily stopping eating and drinking; depression relief; and spiritual counseling.

To correct such lapses as may occur, medical schools have modified their curricula to prepare future physicians to be able to help better in end-of-life decisions. A new specialty of geriatric care is being implemented in both medical education and hospital and nursing practice. Federal funding has been increased for Medicare to pay doctors and specialists for counseling as part of programs for medically assisted dying. (See chapter 5 for further discussion.)

Any early lapses to prepare terminally ill patients with sufficient end-of-life counseling to make wise decisions for their end-of-life care has been corrected.

Abuse for Financial Gain

Some elderly patients, others with limited mental capacity, members of minority groups, or those with significant financial assets may be deprived of a longer life through being coerced to choose medically assisted dying by family members or others who stand to gain financially from a patient's estate. To prevent this and ensure the procedure has been followed correctly, with no coercion, one witness to the terminally ill patient's signing the request for a lethal drug must have no interest in the patient's estate.

When All Attempts at Medically Assisted Dying Fail

An overlooked benefit of medically assisted dying laws is that they offer a compassionate alternative to suicide. Many of the roughly 44,000 suicides that occur each year in the United States might be avoided by the individuals' taking part in medically assisted dying. In an example discussed later in this chapter, a resident of Washington, which had enacted a medically assisted dying law that became effective in 2009, was in a Catholic hospital that denied him a lethal drug to end his suffering. The man was in excruciating pain and pleaded for the help to which he was legally entitled. The help was denied, and the man then shot and killed himself. In other cases, terminally ill patients had begun the process for obtaining lethal drugs under their state's medically assisted dying law but failed to complete the multi-step process before dying of their illness.

An unfortunate scenario that has played out many times is the death of an elderly patient in terrible and prolonged agony who repeatedly begged a spouse or adult child to help them die — and the other could finally no longer resist the pleas and killed their beloved husband, wife, father or mother by smothering, poison, or other means. In the legal cases that followed, the killer was often judged guilty of a misdemeanor rather than a crime such as murder and was paroled rather than jailed. Allowing a patient to end their suffering and allow them a compassionate and dignified death by a law that legalizes medically assisted dying is simply much better than suicide.

H.Con.Res.80 – 115th Congress (2017-2018)

A comprehensive statement of the many reasons advanced by the political opposition against medically assisted dying is contained in a joint bipartisan resolution of the House of Representatives and Senate of the 2017-2018 Congress of the United States. It is identified as "H.Con.Res.80 – 115th Congress (2017-2018)," abbreviated as H. Con. Res. 80. Its full text is given in Appendix A.

The resolution was introduced in the House of Representatives on September 26, 2017, almost twenty years after the Death with Dignity Act was enacted in the state of Oregon. By then, six other states and the District of Columbia had enacted similar medically assisted dying laws, the laws had already aided roughly four thousand terminally ill patients to end their suffering with dignity, and the Supreme Court had ruled that states had the right to pass such laws. Their record of success is discussed in Chapter 2. It was overlooked or simply ignored by the authors of H.Con.Res.80 – 115th Congress (2017-2018).

The joint resolution of the 115th Congress against medically assisted dying is largely a collection of misunderstandings, errors, unsupported claims, and biases that are held by opponents. It provides a convenient and comprehensive summary of issues that have been voiced over and over by legislators and political activists opposed to medically assisted dying laws — and have been shown to be false and unjustified. Let us recognize it for just that.

Appendix A reproduces the full text of H. Con. Res. 80. It includes an introductory clause, 22 "Whereas" clauses, and a final clause with the resolution itself. Each of the 24 sections is followed by a rebuttal, and Appendix A ends with some concluding comments.

RELIGIOUS OPPOSITION

When we speak of religion in what follows, we define religion as the belief and worship of a superhuman controlling power – that is, a personal god or deity responsible for the creation of the universe in which we live. Active participation in a religion is living a life that follows the moral principles of the chosen religion, as they were revealed by its founder and possibly enlarged or modified later by the religion's prelates or leaders. Founders of religions sometimes claim having had revelations of a god's will directly or through earlier prophets or "wise men" who themselves claimed to have had personal contacts from the deity.

A religion's rules of conduct or *modus operandi* are codified in a set of commandments, often composed by later leaders after the founder's death. There are also rituals and sacraments or holy orders that advocatess of a religion must follow or participate in.

In the United States and the Western culture, the leading religion is Christianity. It includes the Roman Catholic Church, various Protestant sects that splintered off from it during and after the Protestant Reformation (1517-1648), several Revivalist religions (such as those in the Southern "Bible Belt" of southeastern and some central parts of the United States), Quakers, and other protestant sects

Buddhism, Taoism, Confucianism, and Shinto are followed by a minority in the United States. They are strictly *not* religions because they lack a superhuman god or deity. Instead, they are traditions, philosophies, or simply ways of life based on such humanistic or rationalistic principles as charity, love, humility, tolerance, forgiveness, friendship, and — above all, respect for others.[3]

These principles are guides for social or ethical conduct that were learned from mortals rather than revealed or taught by a deity who descended from a mythical heaven and assumed human form. They are also called virtues, and they are endorsed by Catholicism and other Christian religions. Their emphasis on man and mankind rather than on a superhuman deity is the essence of what began in Europe during the Enlightenment or Age of Reason. They are embodied in the principles of secular morality that are imbedded in our social and political system of democracy.

We might reasonably believe that the historical Jesus was, in fact, a mortal human like Buddha and Confucius, and that he was much respected and widely followed for his teachings of charity, love, tolerance, forgiveness and so forth, That is, the essence of Jesus' teachings is much like the natural philosophies of Buddha, Confucius, Taoism and Shinto.

There are several schools of Buddhism and Confucianism, and they have a more tolerant view of medically assisted dying and euthanasia than those of the Catholic Church. For example, the Tibetan Dalai Lama himself has held that "In the event a person is *definitely* going to die and he is either in great pain or has virtually become a vegetable, and prolonging his existence is only going to cause difficulties and suffering for others, the termination of his life may be permitted according to Mahayana Buddhist ethics."[4]

A major difference between religious morality and secular morality lies in the enforcement of the moral principles rather than the principles themselves, which are similar. For religious morality, teaching and enforcement are the job of a religious leader such as the pope and, at the lower levels, archbishops, bishops, and priests, assisted by religious brothers, monks, and nuns and by their churches, religious schools and teachers. For secular morality, as practiced in the United States, it is the job of government officials elected by voters at federal, state, county, and municipal levels and by systems of public schools and teachers to instruct and systems of courts of law and police to enforce.

Neither the church nor our government do a perfect job of practicing or enforcing religious or secular laws. That is the cause of much of our society's failure and divisiveness. We can and should do better.

OPPOSITION OF
THE ROMAN CATHOLIC CHURCH

Major opposition to medically assisted dying has been and continues to be voiced by prelates of the Roman Catholic Church. Pope Francis has himself denounced it as a "false sense of compassion," and a sin against God and creation.[5] It is also said to be a violation of the sanctity and inviolability of human life. An example of this opposition provided in the following episode.

On June 16, 2011, while a coalition of concerned citizens in Massachusetts was gathering signatures to place a voters' initiative on the 2013 state ballot to make medically assisted dying legal, the United States Conference of Catholic Bishops released a document titled "To Live Each Day with Dignity: A Statement on Physician-Assisted Suicide." This was the first time the full body of bishops issued a statement regarding the issue of medically assisted dying.

The Bishops' manifesto began by recognizing that many people fear the dying process today. As the document states: "They are afraid of being kept alive past life's natural limits by burdensome medical technology. They fear experiencing intolerable pain and suffering, losing control over bodily functions, or lingering with severe dementia. ... They worry about being abandoned or becoming a burden on others."[6]

From these opening observations, the bishops' position drifts into five full pages of questionable theological dogma that forms the basis of their opposition to medically assisted dying. The gist of their opposition is contained in the following exchange between a newspaper reporter and the associate director of the bishops' conference.

The reporter asked, "Is it immoral to end a dying life? Even if it is one's own?"

"If what?" the associate director pointedly asked.

"If it's one's own life," the reporter repeated.

"It isn't one's own," was the response.[7]

This view of the sanctity and inviolability of the human body — that is, the belief that the human body was created in the image of God and is the property of the Creator — is part of the belief in supernatural beings (i.e., a deity of three persons and multitudes of angels and devils) of Catholic dogma.

Moreover, bishops and other Catholic prelates claim that it is their divinely-given right of authority to claim your body belongs to that Creator and to decide for you what that deity expects and commands from you — under pain of eternal damnation if you act in opposition. This and other dogmatic views are the basis of their opposition to divorce, contraception, abortion, and gay rights, for example, as well as to medically assisted dying.

Bishops and other members of the Catholic hierarchy admonish terminally ill Catholics to accept their end-of-life pain and distress as what they call "redemptive suffering." In explanation of "redemptive suffering," the Bible teaches that when we are made to suffer, it is for our own consolation and salvation and to bring us closer to Christ, who suffered for us (2 Corinthians, 1:5-6).

Despite this admonition, many nominal Catholics (perhaps the majority) are in favor of laws that legalize medically assisted dying. Many who proclaim themselves Catholics and attend Mass, go to confession, receive communion, and practice much of what their Church preaches — have been divorced and remarried, practice birth control, have had abortions, accept gay marriage, and other practices condemned by the Church. They also perform good works and practice love, tolerance, charity, and forgiveness as Christ and others taught, and they approve or favor the legalization of medically assisted dying.

Some specific rights to our bodies are controversial — for example, a woman's rights to abortion, the right to life of a seriously defective fetus or one that is the result of rape. Women's rights are a point of contention even with Catholic nuns, some of whom have marched in protest against their treatment as inferiors in the Church hierarchy, much as working women have protested their inferior positions and harassment in corporate hierarchies.

For many years, the Church's teachings that a person's body belonged to a deity extended even beyond death – that sinners who died without confessing their serious or mortal sins would live forever in the torments of hell. Today, many of us carry cards in our wallets or purses that allow our eyes and other organs to be removed from our corpses and implanted in the bodies of others so that they can enjoy a more satisfying life, or that allow our cadavers to be used for medical research that will benefit others. Such practices are another way of honoring the sanctity of the human body, as well as heart-felt compassion for others.

While many of us accept that there is a god, in the sense that there is a primal, creative force for the world in which we find ourselves, we do not believe in a superhuman or personal god, as viewed by Christian/Catholic, Jewish, Islamic, and other religions. We simply admit that we do not know the nature and characteristics of the primal force that created the universe, and it is presumptuous to suppose that we can know its mind or any intent it might have for us. You can name it Father Time, Mother Nature, The Big Bang, or God, as you wish. Perhaps astrophysicists and other scientists will someday unravel its mystery and character. Until then, we recognize no logical basis for knowing and understanding a personal deity.

We mean no disrespect, but we hold it preposterously arrogant to assert that man was created in the image and likeness of God, as suggested by a literal belief in the biblical statement in the book of Genesis that "in the image of God has God made man." (Genesis, 9:6).

We respect Jesus, Buddha, Confucius and, more recently, Mother Teresa, Pope Francis and others, both male and female, who have preached and practiced doctrines of love, charity, tolerance, and forgiveness as good human beings, much of whose lives are worthy of imitation.

We question some teachings of church rule and control over others that was expressed in the decades following Jesus' death. The apostle Paul, in his letters to the Romans, admonishes the people to obey Rome's rulers. He asserts that the authority of monarchs, popes. and other rulers in the broad sense is given to them by god, and that to disobey the god-given authority of rulers is to disobey god itself. That is the gist of the bishops' manifesto discussed earlier. That is what is meant by "the divine right of kings." It is expressed by the observation that "Religion is regarded by the common people as true, by the wise as false, *and by rulers as useful*."[8]

Our founding forefathers were well aware of the apostle Paul's admonitions and "the divine right" of kings. They recognized the danger of adding religious authority to the secular authority of rulers and established the separation of church and state.[9] This separation was designed to keep from mixing religious authority with the democratic principles expressed as "the rights of man," as set forth in the Preamble of our Constitution. Therefore, they added the following words, "Congress shall make no law respecting an establishment of religion or prohibiting the free exercise thereof ..." to the first Amendment of the Constitution of the United States.

Our Supreme Court has upheld the right of Catholic popes, bishops, and lesser religious prelates to preach what they wish and to admonish members of their congregations and dioceses to follow so long as it is consistent with the separation of Church and State. It has also upheld the right of states to enact laws that give their residents the right to medically assisted dying.

Each of us has the right to practice and preach a religion of our choice, or to practice no religion, so long as we obey our nation's laws. And each of us has the right to avail ourselves of medically assisted dying in states where it is legal, and to advocate for its legalization in states where it is not.

The Sanctity and Inviolability of Human Life

The official position of the Catholic Church regarding the sanctity of life and the human body, as in the statements noted earlier, has been remarkably elastic. The commandment "Thou shalt not kill" has been stretched many ways over the past centuries to condone improper or controversial Church practices. It was ignored in justifying such wars as the following:

- The Crusades, which were a series of religious wars sanctioned by the Roman Catholic Church to suppress paganism and heresy, to resolve conflicts, and/or to gain political and territorial advantage (1095-1510).[10]
- The Guelph and Ghibelline Wars, which were fought between factions allied to Roman Catholic Popes and those allied with the Holy Roman Emperors for political and religious power (1215-1392).[11]
- The Inquisitions, which were a series of institutions from the 12th century to the present that was sanctioned by the Roman Catholic Church to suppress religious dissent and heresies (1209-1834).[12]
- The Thirty Years War, which was fought between various Catholic and Protestant states and factions, It started as a religious war between various Catholic and Protestant city-states in Germany, and it expanded through much of Central Europe to become one of the most destructive conflicts in human history. It caused some eight million fatalities from military engagements and to related violence, famine, and plague (1618-1648).[13]

While opposed to abortion and protective of the life of unborn fetuses, the Catholic Church has stretched its beliefs in the sanctity and inviolability of the human body to the use of castrati in church choirs (1550-1902).[14] The castrati were adult males who had been castrated while pre-pubescent boys to preserve their high-pitched voices. They were used as substitutes for women, whom church law forbade to speak or sing in church during mass and other rites, to provide the high-pitched voices needed for hymns. The young boys who survived castration underwent years of singing and music lessons so that, after they had matured, they could sing the high treble parts of hymns. They were used in church choirs in the Vatican and many other churches in Europe for over three centuries.

At its peak around 1720 – 1730, more than 4,000 young boys were castrated each year. Many died as a result of the operation to remove their testicles. Church laws have changed, and women now have the right to sing in the choirs of Catholic churches during mass and other rites.

All the above practices, which were undertaken to preserve and display the power of religious morality, caused the deaths of millions of innocents, many under the most painful of conditions.

In more recent time, there have been widespread cases of chid seexual abuse by Catholic priests, nuns and members of religious orders. The abused were mostly boys but also girls between the ages of 11 and 14, with some as young as three years old.[15]

Thankfully, religious morality has been largely replaced by secular morality during the Enlightenment, also called the Age of Reason. It took place from the mid-16th to early-18th centuries (i.e., during what has been abbreviated as "the long 17th century"). It followed the Renaissance, and it began as the Catholic Church's dominance in religious morality was weakened by the Protestant Revolution that began in the early 16th century.

Despite the opposition of Catholic prelates, there is strong support for medically assisted dying among Catholic laity. This includes strong support among Catholics who are ethnically Hispanics and Latinos and who now comprise about 34 percent of the Catholic population of the United States. It is also shown by the support that has been given by their leaders (e.g., Dolores Huerta, Mauricio Ochman, and Jorge Ramos) and by such organizations as the National Hispanic Council on Aging, the Hispanic-Health Network, and the Latino Commission of AIDS to laws for medically assisted dying dying.[16]

African-Americans also strongly support medically assisted dying. For example, in Washington, D.C., a heavily African America city, all but one African-American members of the city council voted in favor of the city's "Death with Dignity Act of 2015."[17]

The Catholic church is an accepted part of our American society, and it does much good. Manhy members of the Catholic Church have helped in caring for the sick and dying and in promoting social justice for the poor and unfortunate. Pope Francis has become a welcome champion for love, charity, tolerance, and the respect for the dignity of others that are the essence of what Jesus Christ peached.

Like participation in medically-assisted dying, participation in religious beliefs and practices is a choice. The choice for medically assisted dying should be allowed to terminally ill patients, their doctors, and the pharmacists who dispense doses of lethal medications. No one is being forced to do what they oppose, do not believe in, or do not wish to do. Religion itself is a choice. Our nation's Constitution gives each of us the freedom to practice whatever religion we wish, as well as the freedom to profess no religion whatsoever.

The Sanctity and Inviolability of Life

In his book *The Future of Assisted Suicide and Euthanasia*, Neil Gorsuch, who became an Associate Justice of the United States Supreme Court in April 2017, asserts his belief in what he names "the inviolability of life principle," and he argues that it provides a secure argument against medically assisted dying.[18] It is the same argument as that advanced by the Union of American Bishops, as discussed earlier.

In ethics, which refers to the moral principles that establish what is right and what is wrong and that govern a person's behavior or how one conducts themselves, the inviolability of life principle asserts that life has values that require respect and care and are not to be violated. This respect for the life of another is part of the *secular* theory of morality, which is the basis of our social and political system of democracy which, in turn, is based on a belief in man and mankind. Secular morality is based on the ownership of one's own body and on our social contract with others, which teaches us to do unto others as we would have them do unto us.

Alternatively, the respect for life is also part of the *religious* theory of morality, which is based on the belief in a superhuman personal deity that claims possession and control over each human life and gives it a holy or sacred value.

The rules of secular authority are defined and enforced by people, either directly by themselves or indirectly by delegates, and they are enforced by people elected or appointed do so. The rules of Catholic religious authority are defined by Popes and synods of bishops and other prelates who claim to speak with divine authority in matters of faith and morals, and they are enforced by a system of commandments, self-confession of trespasses, and personal atonement administered by parish priests.

The inviolability of life principle is a basic belief or ethic that is part of our social and political system of democracy. It refers to how we treat one another as equals in many respects. It basically refers to life's being very important and deserving respect.

Though some may disagree, it can also include respect for the dying wishes of mentally competent adults who are terminally ill and suffering — and who wish to die on their own terms, surrounded by family and friends, and with both their autonomy over their life and its dignity intact. It includes compassion for those who deeply feel their loss of autonomy and their loss of control over bodily functions. Respecting their loss is a much better recognition of the sanctity and inviolability of human life than a rigid insistence on keeping such individuals alive against their wish to end their distress and suffering, even if it means their death. It is much better than the belief that one's body belongs to a supernatural deity or some unknowable creative force that is said to claim ownership of our bodies and that judges our final suffering to be due payment for some trespass against the deity.

Though the inviolability of life principle applies in both secular and religious morality, how it is correctly observed can vary with the conditions under which it is applied, and the laws concerning its pairing with death can be very controversial and inconsistent. Thus, although a competent adult does have a constitutional right to demand the removal of distressful life-support healthcare that's essential to sustain their life, even though its removal will result in their death, they do *not* have the constitutional right to have access to medical means, such as a dose of a lethal drug they can ingest to remove their distresses but will result in their death. Though both examples — the first for removing a medical tool or technique and the second for using a medical tool or technique — would have the same benefit of removing distress but cause the individual's death, current United States law allows the first but not the second as a constitutional right. The second is a right only in states that have enacted legislation to legalize it. (See the cases discussed in Chapter 4 for a few examples of the law's conditions for involving the inviolability of life principle.)

Justice Gorsuch appears to argue that the inviolability of life principle is a basically good principle that is to be followed whatever the circumstances. He insists that "intentional acts by private persons against basic goods, including life, are categorically wrong."[19] Over-and-over, he describes life as "a basic good" and denounces medically assisted dying laws (which he improperly calls "assisted suicide") as violations of the "sanctity of life" or the "inviolability-of-life principle" and "categorically wrong." In the sense used by Gorsuch, the term "categorically wrong means "absolutely, unconditionally, or without qualification"; that is, something is always wrong, without exception, or for which there are never, never any extenuating circumstances or conditions that would make them correct.

Gorsuch chatters on, positing one situation after another, and asking "But is the notion of noninstrumental, the concept of categorical rights and wrongs, altogether foreign in our lives? I would suggest that the answer is no. Don't we, at least sometimes, honor our family or members or friends, the works of nature or art, or those older and wiser or younger and more vulnerable, not for any instrumental or contingent usefulness they may have, but simply out of respect for their innate value?"[20]

The essential basic question to be answered here is whether or not a competent, terminally ill adult patient who complies with all the caveats of medically assisted dying laws to prevent abuses has the right to die by choosing to ingest a lethal drug. And though Justice Gorsuch and the Catholic Church would answer "No" to such a choice, this writer and likely most readers and others would say "Yes." But if you choose to say "No," it's your choice and you should be free to make it. And please don't impose your choice on those of us who don't share your beliefs.

Suicide: An Ugly Alternative to Medically Assisted Dying

In the absence of medically assisted dying, many terminally ill individuals end their suffering by suicide — by shooting themselves with guns, by jumping from the upper floors of tall buildings, by ingesting a cache of sleeping pills, by refusing food and water, or by asphyxiating themselves by hanging or the "bag method.". Such methods are wide open to abuses, either by individuals seeking their own deaths or by others who encourage them to commit suicide in order to profit from their deaths. Medically assisted dying laws provide a compassionate alternative to suicide with safeguards to prevent abuses.

According to data provided by the American Foundation for Suicide Prevention (AFSF), suicide is the tenth leading cause of death in the United States, and the current annual rate is estimated aa roughly 44,000 suicides per year.[21] While this number is the most accurate we have, AFSF estimates the actual number is higher because of the underreporting that results from the stigma surrounding suicide. And for every successful suicide, there are said to be an average of 25 attempts.

Suicide rates vary with age. The AFSF has measured the annual rates of suicide by the number per 100,000 persons in 10-year groups. The highest suicide rate in 2016 was 19.72 suicides per 100,000 for middle-age adults between 45 to 54 years old. Except for this group, suicide rates increased with age. The second highest rate was 18.98 suicides per 100,000 for those 85 years or older. Young adults aged 15 to 24 had a suicide rate of 13.15 per thousand.

The American Foundation for Suicide Prevention estimates that suicides cost the United States $69 billion annually. Many individuals who commit suicide are struggling with mental illness and could be helped by psychiatric counseling. Unfortunately, such care is not always available because of its cost. Much of this cost could be eliminated, or diverted to better uses, if more states legalized medically assisted dying.

The benefits, or "beneficial consequences," of passing laws for medically assisted dying far outweigh the consequences that individuals and society are paying for not having such laws.

OPPOSITION OF CATHOLIC HOSPITALS

Catholic hospitals now comprise ten of the 25 largest healthcare networks in the United States. They are allowed by law to deny providing abortions, medically assisted dying, or any other healthcare service that requires them to act in a manner that is inconsistent with their religious beliefs or teachings. However, although their staffs of administrators, physicians, nurses, and other healthcare providers can deny such *services*, they are required by law to *volunteer full information to alternate care and help where a patient seeking such services or help can obtain them.*

The religious principles that administrators, staff, and visiting physicians must practice are codified in the Ethical and Religious Directives (ERD) for Catholic Health Care Services, which have date from 1921. Beginning in 1948, they have been published by the United States Conference of Catholic Bishops.

The latest edition of the Ethical and Religious Directives for Catholic Health Care Services was issued November 17, 2009. Its Directive Number 60 opposes participating in euthanasia or assisted suicide (i.e., their names for medically assisted dying). In explaining the Catholic church's opposition to medically assisted dying and its acceptance of suffering, Directive 61 comments "Patients experiencing suffering that cannot be alleviated should be helped to appreciate the Christian understanding of redemptive suffering"[22] — that is, as the Bible teaches, when we are made to suffer, it is for our own

74

consolation and salvation (2 Cor. 1:5, 6) and for bringing us closer to Christ, who suffered for us.

Bishops have some leeway in interpreting and applying the Directives, which Catholic hospitals in their dioceses must follow. They have ruled out medically assisted dying for violating principles of the Catholic religion, and they will not allow their physicians and other providers to provide it, even for those who are not Catholics and do not share their beliefs.

Catholic hospitals refuse to provide many services to women which are legal, such as *emergency abortions due to pregnancy complications, as required by federal law.*

In short, although Catholic hospitals are funded by federal and state agencies, they often violate state or federal laws — and have done so for many years.

An Example of Abuse: In 2014, in Washington State, where medically assisted dying had been made legal in 2008, a hospice patient who was terminally ill with brain cancer repeatedly begged for the aid to which he was legally entitled as a resident of Washington in order to end his life and avoid excruciating pain. However, he was in a hospice affiliated with Providence Health & Services,[23] which is a large network of Catholic healthcare facilities. His physician and other medical professions assigned to his care refused — refused not only to provide the aid themselves. *but even refused to provide information or referrals to other places that might help him, as required by law.* They apparently understood that, as a matter of the hospital's policies, they would be fired if they offered the patient a referral to another facility or a physician who would provide medically assisted dying.

The man eventually solved the refusal of the hospice to provide help by climbing into a bathtub, where he shot himself with a gun.

The Case of Sister Margaret McBride: In November 2009, a 27-year-old woman who was eleven weeks pregnant with her fifth child was admitted to St. Joseph's Hospital and Medical Center, a Catholic facility in mid-town Phoenix, Arizona. The hospital was owned by Catholic Healthcare West, a unit of Dignity Health, and staffed by nuns of the order of the Sisters of Mercy. The pregnant woman was diagnosed as gravely ill with "right heart failure," and doctors advised that she had close to a 100 percent chance of dying if she continued her pregnancy. The patient was too ill to be moved to another hospital for surgery. According to the U.S. Catholic Church's ethical guidelines, the mandated solution would be to let both the mother and the unborn fetus die.[24,25] This would have left the woman's four children without their mother.

A way out of the dilemma was found in Directive 47 of the Church's ethical guideline, which under some circumstances allowed procedures that could kill the fetus while saving the mother. The woman consented to an abortion, and her family, her physicians, and the hospital's Ethics Committee agreed to her choice. Sister Margaret McBride, a Sister of Mercy who was Vice President of the hospital and a member of the hospital's ethics committee, approved an abortion, and the woman survived.

The abortion came to the attention of Bishop Thomas J. Olmsted of the Phoenix diocese. He declared Sister Margaret to be excommunicated automatically for allowing an abortion to be performed at a Catholic hospital. On December 21, 2010, Bishop Olmsted announced that the Roman Catholic Diocese of Phoenix was severing its affiliation with Saint Joseph's Hospital because the hospital's management refused to promise not to perform abortions in the future.[26] The implication was that the Church preferred to allow nature to take its course, which would have resulted in the death of the mother of four as well as likely the one unborn.

A public outcry followed. Doctors approved what Sister McBride had done and described her as saintly. Others pointed to the Church's double standard. No pedophile priests have been excommunicated, and bishops have protected those found guilty rather than defrocking them. Despite papal opposition, the Church's scandal over pedophile priests continues.

Sister Mary resigned her position at the hospital at the Bishop's request. She confessed her action, and in December 2011 her excommunication was lifted. She has since rejoined the hospital in another position, and she is in good standing with the Sisters of Mercy.

Secular Morality

Secular morality is an alternative to religious morality. As religious morality is more and more challenged as unsatisfying and not supported by either logic or science, it is being replaced by secular morality.

Religious morality had been part of the rule of ancient kingdoms. From the time of the Roman Empire, it was based on hereditary monarchs and elected Popes of the Catholic Church and concepts such as "the Divine Right of Kings." Monarchs responsible for temporal rule and Popes responsible for spiritual rule joined forces, each supporting the other except during the many divisive periods of war caused by periodic corruption, greed, and lusts for power, when monarchs opposed popes and popes opposed monarchs. Most people were serfs bound to the lands of monarchs and lesser princes. They had no voice in government, raised food to serve those in authority, and bore the brunt of suffering during periods of warfare.

The development of modern secular morality in Europe began during the Enlightenment, also known as the Age of Reason. It took place during the "long 17th century" – that is, from the late 16th century to the early 18th century. It gave voice to each nation's populace. Over several centuries, it gradually replaced the ancient concept of joint rule by hereditary monarchs and elected Popes with social and political systems based on democracy and "the Social Contract," which is succinctly worded as "Do unto others as you would have them do unto you."

The basis of secular morality is summarized in the following two lines of Alexander Pope's *An Essay on Man.*

> "Know then thyself, presume not god to scan.
> The proper study of Mankind is man."[27]

Or, as it was alternately expressed, the Age of Reason was a time when the Fatherhood of God was replaced by the Brotherhood of Man.

Secular morality is known by various names, each of which emphasizes different aspects, views or forms that focus on man and mankind, such as:

• **Humanism**:[28] Humanism emphasizes the values and the means or agency of humans, either individually or collectively. It asserts the ability of humans to improve the lives of individuals and their society and organizations by using human knowledge, reason, logic, creativity, and ingenuity to plan and carry out actions. Humanism is opposed to submitting blindly to authority, religious dogma, or tradition, or to sinking into cruelty and brutality.

Humanism was the intellectual basis of the Renaissance (14th to early 16th centuries) and an impetus for the Enlightenment or Age of Reason that followed (mid 16th to early 18th centuries).

Early humanism began from the concept of Roman *humanitas,* a Latin noun meaning human nature, civilization, and kindness; that is, what makes us human, different from savage beasts. It sprang from the rediscovery of classical Greek philosophy, such as that of Protagoras (c/ 490 - 420 BCE), who said that "Man is the measure of all things."

Humanism is centered on humankind (i.e., human needs, interests, and abilities) rather than the supernatural. Humanism emphasizes critical thinking and evidence (i.e., rational and subject to verification by experience) over religious dogma and superstition. It focuses on humans and mankind in relation to one another and to the world. It has influenced and become manifest in art, architecture, literature, politics, and science.

- **Freethinking**: Freethinking (aka Freemasonry) holds that understanding life and truth should be formed on the basis of knowledge, reason, logic, and empiricism rather than authority, tradition, revelation, or religious dogma.

  Freethinking and Freemasonry were both feared by the Catholic Church for aiding or encouraging individuals to think for themselves and develop ideas and beliefs that opposed those of the Church. The Church branded individuals with such ideas as heretics and their beliefs as heresies. During the Inquisitions, more than one thousand individuals branded as heretics were burned alive at the stake for espousing what the Catholic Church regarded as heresies.

- **Consequentialism**: Consequentialism holds that the consequences of one's conduct are the ultimate basis for any judgment about the rightness or wrongness of that conduct. Consequentialism as a theory of the right holds that actions are right insofar as they promote good. However, since actions can have bad as well as good consequences, promoting good implies that an action's good outweighs its bad, including the bad of any unintended consequences.

  The good consequence of medically assisted dying is to shorten or eliminate the suffering of terminally ill patients and their families and close friends. It also replaces a dismal death with an opportunity for a final celebration of life with family and friends. And it might also avoid the consequences of an ugly suicide. Avoiding any bad consequences of medically assisted dying depends on following a rigid procedure for qualifying a terminally ill patient to receive a lethal drug that can be ingested to end the patient's life.

- **Utilitarianism**: Utilitarianism states that the best action is the one that maximizes utility, usefulness, or well-being. It is a version of consequentialism. A sub-branch of Utilitarianism known as Utility Theory uses mathematical models and algorithms to optimize the results of business decisions. A difficulty of utilitarianism is that of assigning utility values to each of the costs and consequences.

Secular morality is the basis for our social and political system of democracy. Its principles and teachings are well expressed by the Preamble of our nation's Constitution, which is the supreme law of the United States and reads as follows:

"We, the People of the United States, in order to form a more perfect Union, establish justice, insure domestic tranquility, provide for the common defense, promote the general welfare, and secure the blessings of liberty to ourselves and our posterity, do ordain and establish this Constitution for the United States of America."[29]

These words are codified in the Constitution itself, and in the laws that have been enacted by Congress, by State legislatures, and by County and Municipal governments to implement and support the Constitution. This includes the 27 amendments to the Constitution, the first ten of which are collectively known as the Bill of Rights. Together with the Fourteenth Amendment, the Bill of Rights guarantee each of us with specific inalienable rights, It also requires us to respect those same rights for others.

Consequentialism and Medically Assisted Dying

Justice Neil Gorsuch of the Supreme Court of the United States has used the form of secular morality known as consequentialism to express a conservative view of medically assisted dying in his book *The Future of Assisted Suicide and Euthanasia*.[30] Gorsuch's book was published by Princeton University Press in 2006, eight years after the implementation of the state of Oregon's Death with Dignity Act. It is used by Justice Gorsuch in a rather muddled attempt to justify his opposition to medically assisted dying.

Justice Gorsuch views human life as a "basic good," which is to be preserved by whatever means necessary and must never be ended by any sort of intervention. That is a rather specious argument — though it lacks real merit, it is superficially plausible but can be wrong as well as correct, depending on conditions and other possibilities, how one interprets them, and the intent or bias of the one advancing the argument or arguing its rightness.

While we agree that there is some truth in asserting human life is basically good, as Justice Gorsuch does, we hasten to add that life is not all good. Much of what is good and what is bad depends on the individual, and there can be a punishment fitted to what is bad or criminal. Other parts depend on the conditions, such as the presence of physical and/or mental pain, from which there should be a choice for release, unless one is a sadist or religious fanatic.

Gorsuch bases his opposition to medically assisted dying on what he struggles to define as a "basic good," as contrasted to what is a "basic bad." Creating such a universal distinction runs into many problems: First, few things in life are either totally good or totally bad. Most are a mix of good and bad. In practice, much depends on how well we control the bad in something in order to take advantage of its good. For example:

- Contraception, divorce, and abortion are a mix of good and bad. Their use is controlled, regulated, or restricted so that the good outweighs the bad.
- Our economic system of capitalism is a basically good system that works well with our social and political system of democracy. But unfettered capitalism leads to the amassing of wealth at the top, as the Scottish economist and philosopher Adam Smith pointed out in his classic 1776 text *The Wealth of Nations*. This in turn, can lead to a badly skewed wealth distribution, followed by the corruption of our democracy by a financial elite at the top — which is essentially the oligarchy of financial elite masquerading under a façade of democracy that we have today. To secure the benefits of capitalism to all citizens, we need to control or regulate its practices so that the wealth *and* power that capitalism creates (based on money at the top working with labor at the bottom to produce goods and services with social value) is more evenly distributed. This is a fundamental responsibility of our government.
- Medically assisted dying, though basically good in its intentions, can be abused. Laws that legalize its practice have caveats and rigid procedures that must be followed so that their good far out-weighs any bad.

Second, whether something is basically good or bad depends on the knowledge, interests, and perspective of whoever is judging it. Things are often judged differently by different judges. The tipping point of the balance between good and bad has changed significantly since the Age of Reason, when the fatherhood of God was replaced by the brotherhood of Man, as explained earlier.

Third, what is basically good or bad depends on the circumstances, conditions, and alternatives from which to choose. Some alternatives that are good under one set of circumstances and conditions can be bad under others. Suicide is no longer a crime, and it no longer carries the strong stigma it once did. In fact, suicide by voluntarily stopping to eat food and drink water has become a socially acceptable means for ending lives of painful suffering or end-of-life distresses.

Fourth, few things exist in isolation by themselves. Almost all are parts of a system of components that are interlinked, so that what happens in one area impacts what happens in others. This linkage is what leads to "the law of unintended consequences" — an important consideration in applying the theory of consequentualism.

Fifth, where actions can have both good benefits and bad consequences or costs, actions should be chosen on the basis of a cost-to-benefit analysis, in which the values of the costs and benefits or consequences may be measured or quantified in terms of their "usefulness to society" rather than dollars and cents. Assigning values or ranking benefits and consequences is a matter of the knowledge, judgment and objectives of the analyst.

The good consequence of medically assisted dying is to shorten or eliminate the suffering of terminally ill patients and their families and close friends. It also replaces the bad consequences of a dismal death with an opportunity for a final celebration of life with family and friends. And it might also avoid the consequences of an ugly suicide. Avoiding any bad consequences of medically assisted dying depends on following a rigid procedure for qualifying a terminally ill patient to receive a lethal drug that can be ingested to end the patient's life.

Sixth, much that can happen is uncertain and a matter of risks and probabilities in both substance and time – that is, in both what might happen and when.

Seventh, some decisions can be deferred until later without significantly impacting their outcomes, while other decisions must be made soon or quickly to obtain a benefit or avoid a catastrophe.

For these reasons, applying consequentialism to justify decisions can be very unsatisfying — as, for example, in the case of a pregnant woman who must choose between ending her own life or aborting an unborn fetus. The consequences of saving one means ending the life of the other. The life of each may be a basic good, but the consequence of choosing life for one is the death of the other.

When applying the logic of consequentialism to decide whether or not to oppose medically assisted dying laws, one should consider the consequences of both having and NOT having such laws. For example, in the absence of medically assisted dying, many terminally ill individuals have ended their suffering by suicide — by shooting themselves with guns, by jumping from the upper floors of tall buildings, by ingesting a cache of sleeping pills, by refusing food and water, or by asphyxiating themselves by hanging. Such methods are wide open to abuses, either by individuals seeking their own deaths or by others who encourage them to commit suicide in order to profit from their deaths.

Medically assisted dying laws provide terminally ill patients with a choice that is theirs to implement. Health management organizations might oppose medically assisted dying because it deprives them from the profits for providing expensive, end-of-life care during the final month or months of terminally ill patients. Heirs to estates might favor medically assisted dying because it hastens the death of a wealthy parent or relative who might be willing and able to pay whatever it costs to keep them alive as long as medically possible.

Medically assisted dying laws provide safeguards to prevent such abuses. They are much better at avoiding abuses that lead to someone's suicide than not having them. They provide a compassionate alternative to suicide for terminally ill patients who are residents of a state where medically assisted suicide has been legalized. (The case of Brittany Maynard discussed in Chapter 2 is a well-publicized example.)

America's suicide rate, currently about 44,000 individuals annually, is due to several causes, including the lack of suitable alternatives. And for every successful suicide, there are an estimated 25 failed attempts. The American Foundation for Suicide Prevention estimates that suicides cost the United States $51 billion annually. Much of this cost could be eliminated, or diverted to better uses, if more states enacted medically assisted dying.[31]

CLOSING COMMENTS

Much of our lives change as we grow older. End-of-life options, such as medically assisted dying laws, allow us to change with it.

The extension of our lives brought about by advances in medical science and other means has introduced both problems and opportunities. Medically assisted dying laws allow us to change for happier and quicker endings to our longer lives rather than accept the pains and agonies of the final stages of life that are otherwise now longer and more intense. The end-of-life options provided by medically assisted dying permit such a change for many. If we live in a jurisdiction where medically assisted dying is legal and we are terminally ill, we can follow the law to acquire a lethal drug. Once we have the lethal drug, we can choose when and how to end our life by ingesting it.

Despite opposition, the bottom line is that the United States Supreme Court has upheld the legality of laws for medically assisted dying in states where they have been enacted. Terminally ill patients who are residents of states where medically assisted dying is legal can choose for themselves whether or not to use the laws to end their suffering. Citizens of states without medically assisted dying laws have the option to continue without them or to change — that is, to legalize such laws either by voter initiatives or through their elected state representatives, or to move to a state that has legalized medi-cally assisted dying. The change is theirs to make.

According to Gallup's annual political poll conducted in May 2018, 72 percent of adult Americans agree that doctors should be able to help terminally ill patients die and only 27 percent are opposed. Politically, according to the same Gallup poll, medically assisted dying is now a bipartisan issue, supported by 80 percent of Democrats, 73 percent of Independents, and 62 percent of Republicans.[32]

Our nation's Constitution gives each of us the freedom to practice the cultural norms that are expressed in our social and political system of democracy and the laws that have been enacted to codify and implement them. It gives each of us, acting together as "We, the people," the right to enact and enforce laws that benefit everyone. It gives each of us the freedom to practice the religion of our choice, or not to practice any religion at all, so long as we act in accord with our nation's laws.

Dozens of religious leaders of many different religions have expressed their support of medically assisted dying. Those of the Roman Catholic Church are conspicuous in voicing a minority position that opposes such laws. Their reason? Your body and its life belong to a supernatural deity that claims them for itself. That 's a belief you have the right to choose for yourself. Others of us believe and choose differently, as is our right.

Medically assisted dying is a personal choice. If you truly believe in the divinity of Jesus Christ and the dogmas preached by Popes and lesser prelates, and if you limit yourself to the moral philosophy of the Catholic Church, or if you are an old-time rigidly conservative opposed to any progressive change when life itself changes, it may not be for you. But please allow the rest of us who believe in secular morality, which is the basis of our social and political system of democracy, the freedom to follow our own choices.

# # # # #

Chapter 4

PHYSICIANS AND HEALTHCARE SYSTEMS

"A physician shall be dedicated to providing
competent medical care, with compassion
and respect for human dignity and rights."[1]

Healthcare is a system of many components.

At the top are physicians, nurses, and hospitals. These are supported by nursing homes, hospices, and specialists as well as various types of care-givers. They are also supported by scientists conducting research to develop new drugs and surgical instruments and by manufacturers of medicines and medical equipment. Many costs are paid by government agencies such as Medicare and Medicaid, by private insurers, and by the patients themselves. Government regulators oversee operations, and courts of law decide legal issues.

Each component of our healthcare system has specific functions and responsibilities for which they are accountable. Politicians and voters may enact laws to legalize medically assisted dying, but the success of such laws depends on how well the many components of the system are managed and work together in support of each other and patients.

A Medscape Ethics Report issued near the end of 2016 showed that in a poll of more than 7,500 U.S. physicians from more than 25 specialties, 57 percent believed medically assisted dying should be available to terminally ill patients.[2] This increase in approval is consistent with the rise from 46 percent in 2010 to 54 percent in 2014. Going back further, to a 2003 study of members of the American Medical Association, only 31 percent then felt that medically assisted dying should be allowed for terminally ill patients. Thus, over a 13-year period, the percentage of physicians favoring medically assisted dying has nearly doubled, rising from a minority of 31 percent to a majority of 57 percent.

The argument for medically assisted dying for patients is well expressed by Marcia Angell, M.D. Dr. Angell wrote that patients, "especially those with cancer or progressive neurologic disorders, may die by inches and in great anguish, despite every effort by their doctors and nurses. Although nearly all pain can be relieved, some cannot, and other symptoms, such as breathlessness, nausea and weakness, are even more difficult to control. In addition, dying sometimes involves great personal indignities, as well as mental distress from the realization that the situation can only grow worse. … I believe it is wrong to require dying patients, against their wishes, to continue on a downhill path of suffering."[3]

PHYSICIANS AND MEDICALLY ASSISTED DYING

Medically assisted dying imposes a new role of helping patients shorten their process of dying alongside a physician's traditional role of healing to avoid dying. This dual role with what seems to be conflicting purposes has understandably caused many physicians to feel uncomfortable, if not bewildered.

This unease has been exploited by those opposed to medically assisted dying. They named medically assisted dying a form of suicide, which commonly carries a stigma attached to it. They combined suicide with adjectives, as in "assisted suicide," which is a definition of euthanasia and is illegal. Still more inflammatory was the designation "physician-assisted suicide." Such basically incorrect and biased terms aroused opposition by both physicians and voters. They cast physicians into roles that fought against their training and ethics and aroused their opposition.

The American Medical Association (AMA), the nation's largest medical group, maintained for a quarter of a century that medically assisted dying is fundamentally incompatible with the physician's role as healer and creates a conflict that is "potentially very damaging" and contrary to AMA

In an article in the *New England Journal of Medicine* in 2012, at a time when voters in Massachusetts were considering an initiative to legalize medically assisted dying, Dr. Lisa Lehmann of the Harvard School of Medicine advanced some compelling reasons for legalizing medically assisted dying. However, because she felt that writing a prescription for a lethal drug was incompatible with her role as a physician and healer, she strongly opposed the initiative's enactment. As a way of getting around her objection, she suggested that either a federal or state agency should be created to write the prescriptions for lethal drugs after receiving directions from the physicians who attended the terminally ill patients. This would distance physicians from what she felt to be a betrayal of their role as healers.[4] This example illustrates how intensely some physicians felt and may still feel about medically assisted dying's being anathema to their traditional role as healers.

Medically assisted dying laws do NOT ask physicians to participate in causing or intending to cause the death of any of their patients. The intent is to end the suffering of patients. The final act that causes death by ingesting a lethal drug is performed by a terminally ill patient alone, without assistance from anyone else, including their attending physician. It is a rational act taken by a mentally competent and terminally ill patient to end their suffering.

In states that have legalized medically assisted dying, a physician's role is (1) to examine patients to ensure they satisfy all conditions for participating, including a prognosis of less than six months to continue living, (2) to complete the required documents, and (3) write prescriptions for the lethal drugs. Physicians do not participate in their patients' obtaining or using the drugs. So long as the law's procedures are followed, physicians are protected from any liability for what their patients do with their lethal drugs.

The various professional societies of physicians and their members are slowly moving away from their long-standing rigid opposition to medically assisted dying, as indicated in the following.

American Medical Association (AMA): At its annual meeting in Chicago on June 11, 2018, the AMA's delegates rejected a recommendation that it continue its opposition to the legalization of medically assisted dying (which AMA persists in mis-labeling "physician-assisted suicide"). Instead, by a vote of 56 to 44 percent, they directed AMA's Council of Ethical and Judicial Affairs (CEJA) to continue to review its past opposition to medically assisted dying and reconsider supporting it or taking a neutral position.[5]

American Academy of Family Physicians (AAFP): In late October 2018, the American Academy of Family Physicians (AAFP), the second largest component society of the AMA with more than 120,000 members, met and adopted a position of "engaged neutrality" for medically assisted dying.

The AAFP delegates who had attended AMA's annual meeting in June, four months earlier, felt that the CEJA report presented there implicitly acknowledged that medical aid-in-dying laws improve end-of-life care, and that such laws encouraged physicians to have the kind of difficult conversations that are too often avoided. The laws were, in their view, opportunities to explore a patient's goals and concerns, to learn what a terminally ill patient found intolerable about their situation, to respond creatively to a patient's needs, and to engage a patient in conversation about all end-of-life care options, including hospice and palliative care.[6]

The American Academy of Family Physicians also rejected using terms like "assisted suicide" or "physician-assisted suicide" in AMA's formal statements or documents.

American College of Physicians (ACP): In September 2017, the American College of Physicians (ACP), the second largest group of physicians, officially reaffirmed (1) its long-held opposition to the legalization of what it continues to call physician-assisted suicide and (2) its professional responsibility to improve the care of dying patients. ACP's president noted that the ACP "acknowledges the range of views on, the depth of feelings about, and the complexity of the issue of physician-assisted suicide. But the focus at the end of life should be on efforts to prevent or ease suffering and on the often-unaddressed needs of patients and families. As a society, we need to work to improve hospice and palliative care, including awareness and access."[7]

Note that the American College of Physicians continues to use the biased term "physician-assisted suicide" for "medically assisted dying." (How difficult it is to change one's mindset.)

National Academy of Medicine (NAM): The National Academy of Medicine (NAM) was founded in 1970 as the Institute of Medicine (IOM). It is now part of the National Academies of Sciences, Engineering, and Medicine. Its name was changed to the National Academy of Medicine on April 28, 2015. It is a volunteer working-group of physicians, scientists and other experts that functions as a nonprofit, non-governmental organization to provide authoritative information and advice concerning health and medical science policies. NAM has taken a neutral position on the legalization of what it labels "physician-assisted death."

A report issued by the Institute of Medicine on September 17, 2014 found that major improvement needed to be made in end-of-life care. Among IOM's key findings were that:
- "Clinicians need to initiate conversations about end-of-life care choices and work to ensure that the decisions made by patients and families are based on adequate information and understanding; and,

- "Incentives, quality standards, and system support are needed to promote improved clinician communication skills and more frequent and productive clinician–patient conversations."[8]

PRINCIPLES OF MEDICAL ETHICS

The medical profession has long subscribed to a body of ethical statements developed primarily for the benefit of their patients. These place physicians' responsibilities to patients first, next to society, then to other health professionals, and finally to themselves. Formal sets of ethical positions have been established by the various national and state medical societies for the guidance of their members. They are standards of conduct which define the essentials of honorable behavior for physicians.

The earliest of the codes of medical ethics was that attributed to the Greek physician Hippocrates (c. 460 - c. 370 BCE). Contrary to popular belief, the phrase "First do no harm" is not part of the Hippocratic oath; instead there is a statement in Greek "I will utterly reject harm and mischief."

The original Hippocratic Oath has been replaced by many modern versions. In all but a few of the more than a hundred medical schools in the United States, graduating medical students use modern versions of the Hippocratic Oath or other medical codes to swear that they will uphold specific ethical standards. The pledge not to "administer a poison to anybody when asked to do so, nor will I suggest such a course," which appears in the translation of the original text of the Hippocratic Oath, has been dropped in modern versions. Less than 10 percent of the codes of ethics used in U.S. medical schools today prohibit euthanasia and abortion.

An early interpretation of the physician-patient relationship is included in the Code of Medical Ethics adopted in 1847 by the American Medical Association. Chapter 1 is entitled "Of the Duties of Physicians to their patients and of the obligations of patients to their physicians." It states that physicians should "unite tenderness with firmness, and condescension with authority, so as to inspire the minds of their patients with gratitude, respect, and confidence." It then adds, "Reasonable indulgence should be granted to the mental imbecility and caprices of the sick."[9]

Another paragraph includes: "[T]he physician should be the minister of hope and comfort to the sick; that, by such cordials to the drooping spirit, he may smooth the bed of death, revive expiring life, and counteract the depressing influence of those maladies which often disturb the tranquility of the most resigned in their last moments. The life of a sick person can be shortened not only by the acts, but also by the words or the manner of a physician. It is, therefore, a sacred duty to guard himself carefully in this respect, and to avoid all things which have a tendency to discourage the patient and to depress his spirits."[10] While physicians were to avoid advising patients of bad news of their condition, their duties included the following: "But he should not fail, on proper occasions, to give to the friends of the patient timely notice of danger when it really occurs; *and even to the patient himself, if absolutely necessary*."[11] (Italics added for emphasis.)

A physician's role with patients seeking the help of medically assisted dying today is much changed from that summarized in the preceding paragraph.

Until rather recently, physicians made decisions on how to treat terminally ill patients without fully discussing their conditions, treatments, and possible outcomes and risks with the patients themselves. Physicians were not encouraged to discuss fully their conditions with terminally ill patients. There was no established practice of informed consent by terminally ill patients to their physician's decisions for treatment. Thus, as pointed out in a well-documented article published in 2007: "The 1940 Code of Ethics of the American Medical Association provided that "a physician should give timely notice of dangerous manifestations of the disease to the friends of patients [while ignoring the patients themselves]."[12]

Patients and their attending physicians are now on a more even footing for sharing their thoughts about problems and treatments. This is a significant change for the better in making end-of-life decisions for terminally ill patients.

Medical Codes of Ethics

The following are the American Medical Association's nine Principles of Medical Ethics. They were first adopted by the AMA in June 1957 and are as revised in June 2001. The principles are given as stated, except for the insertion of three definitions to emphasize the meaning and interpretation of the first principle, and the use of italics for emphasis in principles 1 and 3.[13]

1. A physician shall be dedicated to providing competent medical care, *with compassion and respect for human dignity and rights.* [By definition, "compassion" is a feeling of deep sympathy and sorrow for another who is stricken by misfortune, *accompanied by a strong desire to alleviate the suffering.*

"Respect," in the sense used, means "to honor" (or to act in accordance with). "Human dignity," in a legal sense, is inherent to every human being, inalienable and independent of the state. Human dignity is the most important human right from which all other fundamental rights derive.]

2. A physician shall uphold the standards of professionalism, be honest in all professional interactions, and strive to report physicians deficient in character or competence, or engaging in fraud or deception, to appropriate entities.

3. A physician shall respect the law and *also recognize a responsibility to seek changes in those requirements which are contrary to the best interests of the patient.*

4. A physician shall respect the rights of patients, colleagues, and other health professionals, and shall safeguard patient confidences and privacy within the constraints of the law.

5. A physician shall continue to study, apply, and advance scientific knowledge, maintain a commitment to medical education, make relevant information available to patients, colleagues, and the public, obtain consultation, and use the talents of other health professionals when indicated.

6. A physician shall, in the provision of appropriate patient care, except in emergencies, be free to choose whom to serve, with whom to associate, and the environment in which to provide medical care.

7. A physician shall recognize a responsibility to participate in activities contributing to the improvement of the community and the betterment of public health.

8. A physician shall, while caring for a patient, regard responsibility to the patient as paramount.

9. A physician shall support access to medical care for all people.

DR. JACOB "JACK" KEVORKIAN

For years, it was not uncommon for a physician attending a terminally ill patient who was rational and wanted to die to leave a vial of morphine or other substance within reach of the patient, well aware that the patient might use the material to end their life. Such action exposed physicians to being charged with "aiding, assisting, or encouraging another to end their life," which is defined as a crime in state laws. Understandably, the likelihood of criminal prosecu-tion and the loss of their license to practice medicine overcame the compassion of physicians for their patients and discouraged the practice.

Taking a Stand for Change

Dr. Jacob "Jack" Kevorkian was a physician who "broke rank" with other physicians. He sought to follow the third principle of ethics of the American Medical Association — that is, "to seek changes in those requirements [he saw as] contrary to the best interests of the patient."

Kevorkian is best known for publicly championing the legal right to provide terminally ill patients with the means that patients could themselves use to end their suffering by ending their lives; that is, he advocated making medically assisted dying legal. When his actions to provide patients with the means to end their suffering failed to trigger attention to the end-of-life suffering of countless patients, Kevorkian himself acted directly on a patient to assist the patient's death.

In 1990, Kevorkian helped a 54-year-old woman diagnosed the year before as suffering from Alzheimer's disease to die. Medically assisted dying laws were not then in effect, so his assisting the death of a patient was a crime. Charges of murder were dropped because there were then no laws in Michigan regarding physician or medically assisted dying. In 1991, however, the State of Michigan revoked Kevorkian's medical license, and he was no longer permitted to practice medicine or work with patients.

Between 1990 and 1998, Kevorkian is alleged to have assisted in the deaths of 130 terminally ill people. In many of these cases, Kevorkian assisted by attaching the individual seeking death to a device he had designed and built. The individual then self-administered a lethal drug by pushing a button which released the drug into their bodies and caused their death. In other cases. people wore gas masks into which carbon monoxide was fed from a canister after the individual opened a valve. Between May 1994 and June 1997, Kevorkian was tried but not convicted four times for helping patients end their suffering. In each case, Kevorkian provided the equipment and lethal drug, but the individuals acted on their own to end their suffering.

Near the end of 1998, the same year that the implementation of Oregon's Death with Dignity Act had begun earlier, Kevorkian took more direct action to attract the attention of others.

On September 17, 1998, Kevorkian made a videotape of his administering a lethal injection to Thomas Youk, who was 52 years old and was in the final stages of Lou Gehrig's Disease (aka amyotrophic lateral sclerosis). Youk had given his fully informed consent, and Kevorkian himself administered a lethal injection, whereas all his earlier clients had themselves reportedly completed the process causing their deaths. Youk's family described the lethal injection as a humane act, not murder.

On November 22, 1998, CBS News' "60 Minutes" television program broadcast the videotape Kevorkian had made of Thomas Youk's voluntary euthanasia.

Four months later, on March 26, 1999, Kevorkian was charged with second-degree murder for Youk's death. Because Kevorkian's license to practice medicine had been revoked eight years previously, he was not legally allowed to possess the controlled substance. After a two-day trial, in which Kevorkian represented himself, the Michigan jury found Kevorkian guilty of second-degree homicide, and he was sentenced to 10 to 25 years in prison. He was paroled for good behavior on June 1, 2007 after spending eight years and two and a half months in prison.

Dr. Kevorkian died on June 3, 2011. The epitaph on his tombstone reads, "He sacrificed himself for everyone's rights."

Many of us regard Dr. Jacob "Jack" Kevorkian as a martyr for a just cause — for putting into action the third principle of the American Medical Association's Code of Ethics: "A physician shall respect the law and *also recognize a responsibility to seek changes in those requirements which are contrary to the best interests of the patient.*" [Italics added for emphasis.] He did so in a defiant act that proved futile at the time — but that has ultimately succeeded in getting changes so that medically assisted dying is legal in states that have enacted laws to make it so.

Dr. Kevorkian's legacy is in the changes that have been made to the traditional interface between physicians and their patients. Whether he is judged right or wrong, Kevorkian was a catalyst for enacting medically assisted dying laws. Such laws had long been overdue. They are still opposed by many prelates and members of the Catholic church and by politically conservative representatives in the U.S. Congress and state legislatures, as discussed in Chapter 3.

Kevorkian's Lasting Impact

By coincidence, 1998 was the year of both the television broadcast of the videotape Kevorkian had made of Thomas Youk's voluntary euthanasia on the "Sixty Minutes" program of CBS News and the first year of the implementation of Oregon's Death with Dignity Act. Both actions forced the medical profession and healthcare system to recognize their new role of taking a more active part to end the suffering of terminally ill patients in addition to their traditional role as healers. However, neither physicians nor the rest of the healthcare system were prepared and ready to accept this new role, and it made them uncomfortable when the role was thrust upon them.

The unpreparedness of physicians in 1998 and what needed to be done was later commented on in the book *The Future of Assisted Suicide and Euthanasia* by Neil Gorsuch, who was appointed an Associate Justice of the U.S. Supreme Court in 2017. Gorsuch's comments are based on only the first five years of the implementation of Oregon's DWDA for which data were available from the state's Health Department at the time of his writing — that is, the years from 1998 to 2002 — during which a total of 129 terminally ill patients received and ingested lethal doses to end their process of dying. He summarized his observations as follows: "Thus, while Oregon is often touted as a 'laboratory' or an 'experiment' for whether assisted suicide [sic] can be successfully legalized elsewhere in the United States, Oregon's regulations are crafted in ways that make reliable and relevant data difficult to obtain. Given this, it is unclear whether and to what extent Oregon's experiment, at least as currently structured, will ever be able to provide the sort of guidance needed and wanted by other jurisdictions considering to follow Oregon's lead."[14]

Gorsuch's comments were directed at the unpreparedness of physicians and the healthcare system to implement and manage Oregon's Death with Dignity Act, not at the purpose or essence of the Act itself.

The unpreparedness of the medical profession for medically assisted dying is also discussed in the lengthy and comprehensive report *Dying in America: Improving Quality and Honoring Individual Preferences Near the End of Life* by Dr. Philip A. Pizzo, MD, Dean Emeritus of the Stanford University School of Medicine, et al., which was issued in 2014 by the Institute of Medicine (IOM), which is now the National Academy for Medicine (NAM). The report provides broad support for Gorsuch's comments from the medical profession itself. The committee of physicians and medical experts who prepared the lengthy report found that "improving the quality and availability of social services for patients and their families could not only enhance quality of life through the end of life, but may also contribute to a more sustainable care system."[15]

The report of the IOM (now NAM) lays out a comprehensive approach to improve the physician-patient interface and the system for end-of-life healthcare. It addresses a large part of the shortcomings of the health care system that Dr. Kevorkian had demonstrated against and that Justice Gorsuch observed. Its recommendations are organized into five categories for action. The most important elements of these are condensed below. They illustrate the breadth and scope of the healthcare system that are being addressed:

1. **Delivery of Care**: Government and private health insurers, as well as care delivery systems, need to provide comprehensive treatment and palliative care that is patient and family oriented; that considers their physical, emotional, social, and spiritual needs; and that is delivered by professionals with appropriate expertise and training.

2. **Clinician-Patient Communication and Advance Care Planning**: Competent individuals should participate with physicians in making health care decisions and plans throughout their lives and as they approach death, and they should receive medical and related social services as consistent with their values, goals, and preferences. Quality standards should be developed and integrated into assessments, care plans, and reporting systems.

3. **Professional Education and Development**: Specifications need to be developed for training and certifying or licensing to strengthen the knowledge of palliative care and medical skills of physicians who care for patients with terminal illnesses.

4. **Policies and Payment Systems**: The financing of medical and related social services should be integrated across all federal, state, and private insurance providers. (This is essential if any reforms needed are to be implemented.)

5. **Public Education and Engagement**: The general public needs to have fact-based information that encourages those with serious illnesses to prepare advance care directives that reflect their needs and values. A coordinated effort to do this should involve civic leaders, public health and other government agencies, community

and faith-based organizations, consumer groups, hospitals and other organizations that provide health-care, payers, employers, and professional societies.

LEGAL ASPECTS OF THE PHYSICIAN-PATIENT INTERFACE

The legal aspects of the physician-patient interface remain a conflicted work in progress. Judicial disagreements, split decisions, and appeals are distressingly common.

Informed Consent

The personal autonomy over one's own body is rooted in common law. It is the basis for the right to control one's body, including the right to refuse any unwanted touching of it or any care that an individual does not want. This right was enunciated in the decisions of the two cases summarized in the following.

Union Pacific Railway Company v. Botsford, 1891: Clara L. Botsford, a railroad passenger, sustained permanent injuries to her brain and spinal cord when a berth in a sleeping car fell upon her head. After she sued the railroad for negligence in causing her injuries, the Railroad claimed it was entitled, without her consent, to examine her to determine the extent of her injuries. However, such an examination would have required anesthesia and surgery.

The United States Supreme Court rejected the Railroad's request. It held that there was no authority under either common law or statutory law for the trial court to order such an examination. The court also asserted that: "No right is held more sacred, or is more carefully guarded by the common law, than the right of every individual to the possession and control of his own person, free from all restraint or interference of others, unless by clear and unquestionable authority of law."[16]

Schloendorff v. Society of New York Hospital, 1914: In January 1908, Mary Schloendorff was admitted to the Society of New York Hospital for treating a stomach disorder. After several weeks at the hospital, the house physician diagnosed a fibroid tumor, and a visiting physician recommended surgery. Schloendorff adamantly declined surgery, but she agreed to be examined while anesthetized. During the examination, doctors performed surgery to remove the tumor. Afterwards, gangrene developed in Schloendorff's left arm, which led to amputating some of her fingers. Mary Schloendorff blamed the surgery and filed suit against the hospital.

The case was heard by the New York Court of Appeal. The five judges who participated in the hearing agreed unanimously that the hospital was guilty of medical battery for performing an operation which Schloendorff had opposed. Justice Benjamin Cardozo wrote in the Court's opinion: "Every human being of adult years and sound mind has a right to determine what shall be done with his own body; and a surgeon who performs an operation without his patient's consent commits an assault for which he is liable in damages. This is true except in cases of emergency where the patient is unconscious and where it is necessary to operate before consent can be obtained."[17,18]

Refusal of Artificial Life-Sustaining Treatment

In the 1970s, cases began reaching the courts that involved patients who refused life-sustaining treatments. The first of these to draw attention to the right of a patient in a persistent vegetative state or their representative to order artificial life support to be withdrawn was the case of *In Re: Quinlan*, which reached the New Jersey Supreme Court in 1976.

In re Quinlan, 1976: In 1975, after two days of not eating followed by a night of drinking alcohol and ingesting tranquilizers, 21-year-old Karen Ann Quinlan passed out, stopped breathing for two 15-minute periods, and lapsed into a persistent vegetative state. Her father asked that the medical ventilator that kept Karen alive be removed. Both her primary physician and the Saint Clare's Hospital, a Catholic hospital in Boonton, New Jersey refused to do so. They feared being charged with a homicide death if they removed the ventilator and Karen died. Karen's father then hired attorneys and filed suit in the Superior Court of New Jersey to be appointed his daughter's legal guardian so he could act on her behalf.

When the Superior Court denied his request, Mr. Quinlan appealed the decision to the New Jersey Supreme Court. On March 31, 1976, after the Court authorized him to speak on his daughter's behalf, he ordered the hospital to cease his daughter's artificial ventilation, which the hospital did.

However, Karen Ann surprised everyone when she continued to breathe on her own. She was moved to a nursing home and fed by artificial nutrition for nine more years, until she died from respiratory failure on June 11, 1985.

Karen Quinlan's case is the first major judicial decision to hold that life-sustaining medical treatment may be discontinued in certain circumstances, even if the patient is unable or incompetent to make the decision themselves and the removal of the treatment could end their life. The New Jersey Superior Court's decision made it clear when removing or withholding life support would not constitute homicide or medical malpractice.[19,20]

Cruzan v. Director, Missouri Department of Health, 1990: This was the first "right to die" case heard by the U.S. Supreme Court. It was decided on June 25, 1990. The case was instrumental in creating and promoting the use of advance health directives to avoid legal conflicts over health care decisions.

In Missouri on January 11, 1983, 26-year-old Nancy Cruzan lost control of her car and was thrown into a water-filled ditch, where she landed face-down. She was rescued by paramedics, who found her with no vital signs and resuscitated her. After three weeks in a coma, she was diagnosed as being in a persistent vegetative state, and surgeons inserted a feeding tube for her continuing care.

Five years later, in 1988, Cruzan's parents asked her doctors to remove their daughter's feeding tube. The hospital refused to do so without a court order, since removal of the tube would cause Cruzan's death, for which the hospital and its staff might be held criminally liable.

The Cruzans went to court against the Missouri Department of Health and received a court order to remove the feeding tube. The trial court ruled that Nancy's telling her friends that if she were sick or injured, "she would not wish to continue her life unless she could live at least halfway normally"[21] had effectively authorized withdrawal of life support.

However, the Missouri Department of Health disagreed, holding that the Cruzans had failed to provide clear and convincing evidence of their daughter's wishes. They appealed the trial court's decision to Missouri's Supreme Court. The Missouri Supreme Court agreed with the lower court's decision, holding that without a living will, the Cruzan's had failed to provide clear and convincing evidence of Nancy's wish not to live in a persistent vegetative state. The Cruzans appealed again, and in 1989 the U.S. Supreme Court agreed to hear the case.

In a split 5-4 decision reached on June 25, 1990, the United States Supreme Court upheld the ruling of the Missouri Supreme Court. It found that nothing in the U.S. Constitution prevents the state of Missouri from requiring "clear and convincing evidence" before terminating life-supporting treatment. The court distin-guished between the right to die and the right to refuse life-sustaining care. Its rulings set several important precedents, which are summarized as follows:

- In the majority opinion written by Chief Justice Rehnquist, the Court ruled that under the Due Process Clause of the Fourteenth Amendment to the U.S. Constitution, mentally competent individuals have the right to refuse unwanted medical treatment — even life-sustaining treatments such as mechanical ventilation (i.e., assisted breathing) and artificially provided hydration and nutrition that are essential to sustain their lives.
- Rather than creating a uniform national standard for all states, each individual state has the right to determine its own standards for an individual's right to die and their right to refuse life-sustaining treatments.
- In the absence of a living will or clear and convincing evidence of what an incompetent person would have wanted, a state's interests in preserving life outweigh the right of other individuals to refuse terminal treatment on behalf of an incompetent patient.
- A third party seeking to refuse medical treatment on behalf of an incompetent patient must follow a set of court-ordered rules established by the state of interest.
- The right to die is not a right protected by the U.S. Constitution; that is, an individual does not have a constitutionally protected right to medically assisted dying. That right depends on the laws of their states of residence, and it is not guaranteed by the U.S. Constitution.

Following the Supreme Court's decision, the Cruzans gathered additional evidence supporting their position that Nancy would have wanted her life support withdrawn. The State of Missouri withdrew since the larger constitutional issue of its right to require what it deemed "clear and convincing evidence" had been upheld by the U.S. Supreme Court.

Facing no opposition, the Judge of Missouri's lower court ruled that the new evidence gathered by the Cruzans satisfied the requirement. He issued a court order to remove Nancy's feeding tube, and that was done on December 14, 1990. Nancy Cruzan died on December 26, 1990, eight years after she had entered a persistent vegetative state and been kept alive by artificial means.

In 1996, six years after Nancy Cruzan's death and funeral, her father killed himself.

Cruzan's case attracted national interest. Right-to-life activists and organizations filed seven separate petitions for a court order to reconnect Nancy's feeding tube. After the court refused, nineteen people entered Cruzan's hospital room, tried to reconnect her feeding tube themselves, and were arrested.

The case of *In re Cruzan* established that the right to die or to avail oneself of medically assisted dying is not guaranteed by the U.S. Constitution; instead, it left it for the states to establish their own standards for the right to refuse artificial life support and to determine the legality and conditions for medically assisted dying.

The Cruzan case generated much interest in living wills and advance directives. It set rules for clear and convincing evidence that a third party must satisfy in order to demonstrate that they knew what health care an incompetent patient would want or would refuse.

It also helped create support for the Patient Self-Determination Act (PSDA), which was passed by the U.S. Congress in 1990 and became effective on December 1, 1991. PSDA's purpose is to ensure that patients are informed of their rights regarding decisions about their medical care. It requires hospitals, nursing homes, health maintenance organizations (HMOs), and other health care institutions that receive federal funding to give patients advance-directive information and to explain the right-to-die options available to them under the laws of their states.

Terri Schiavo Case, 1990-2005: In the early morning of February 25, 1990, Theresa Marie "Terri" (nee Schindler) Schiavo collapsed in the apartment she and her husband shared in St. Petersburg, Florida. She had suffered a cardiac arrest. Although she was successfully resuscitated, the lack of oxygen she had suffered caused massive brain damage and left her comatose — that is, in a state of deep unconsciousness.

After two and a half months with no improvement, she was diagnosed as being in an irreversible persistent vegetative state. For the next two years, doctors attempted without success to return Terri to a state of awareness through speech and physical therapy and other experimental therapy.

In 1998, Michael Schiavo, Terri's husband and her legal guardian, argued that his wife would not have wanted long-term artificial life support with no prospect of recovery, and he petitioned the Sixth Circuit Court of Florida to have her feeding tube removed, as the law provided. Terri's parents, however, disputed the diagnosis and her husband's claim of what Terri would have wished, and they insisted that artificial nutrition and hydration be continued. The controversy moved back and forth in the courts, with Terri's husband's asking that the feeding tube be removed and his wife be allowed to die, and her parents' demanding that the tube be kept in so that their daughter could be hydrated and nourished to keep her alive.

On April 24, 2001, Terri's feeding tube was removed for the first time under a court order obtained by her husband. It was reinserted a few days later under a court order obtained by Terri's parents, who alleged perjury by her husband. The controversy continued in the courts.

On February 25, 2005, a County judge again ordered the feeding tube removed. Several appeals and intervention by the federal government followed, during which the federal courts upheld the original decision to remove the feeding tube. On March 18, 2005, the hospice facility disconnected the feeding tube, and Terri Schiavo died two weeks later.

In the seven years between the first and last removals of Terri Schiavo's feeding tube, there were 14 appeals and numerous motions, petitions, and hearings in the Florida courts; five suits in federal courts; four denials by the U.S. Supreme Court to review lower court decisions; demonstrations by both pro-life and right-to-die activists and disability groups; extensive political intervention by the Florida state legislature, the Florida governor Jeb Bush, and the U.S. President George W. Bush; plus a challenge to U.S. law by the Vatican for allowing artificial feeding and hydration to be stopped.

Following Terri Schiavo's death, both her husband and her family wrote books espousing their sides of the case and got involved in activism over the case's larger issues.[22,23]

The Terri Schiavo case established that, depending on individual circumstances, withholding or withdrawing life-sustaining equipment, medicine, or medical procedures is ethical, legal, and medically appropriate. As a general rule, patients with decision-making capacity (or the legally appointed representative of patients without decision-making capacity) can choose to forego any medical intervention, including artificial nutrition or hydration and the use of cardiopulmonary resuscitation. Patients also have the right to receive as much medication as needed to relieve any pain or suffering.

Before deciding whether to withhold or withdraw life-sustaining treatment, physicians should make sure their patients fully understand the alternatives they can choose. Physicians should themselves understand the values and goals for the care of their patients and their families.

CONCLUDING COMMENTS

The medical profession is profoundly changing in response to (1) the increasing duration of individual lives, (2) improvements in medical technology and practices that prolong lives, (3) the changing interface between physicians and their patients, and (4) the legalization of medically assisted dying.

The role of family physicians has changed from solo or small-group practice and community hospitals or clinics to an enormous largely corporatized for-profit industry. Medical schools are in the process of changing the training of physicians. Post-degree physician residencies focus on one or two related specialties. Medical curricula now include classes that teach how to handle end-of-life issues in addition to traditional medical skills and practices to cure illnesses and extend life. Other classes prepare physicians to discuss end-of-life alternatives with patients that consider patients' wishes and desires for peaceful deaths. Geriatric medicine is a new field of specialization, and hospitals have begun departments of geriatric medicine. The medical profession is moving in the right direction.

Medically assisted dying laws are a benefit for both terminally ill patients and their attending physicians. They are a positive benefit to the patients, whether they are among the roughly two-thirds of those who receive and ingest doses of lethal medication to end their dying or the one-third of those who, having had some sense of autonomy restored by possessing lethal drugs, continue their lives until dying of their terminal illnesses or other causes. Medically assisted dying laws protect physicians from prosecution for the help they provide their patients to reduce their suffering and to allow them a dignified death.

As a practical matter, relatively few physicians have written a prescription for a lethal medication under a state medically assisted dying laws. For example, in the first twenty years of experience with Oregon's Death with Dignity Act, less than 1 percent per year of Oregon's roughly 14,000 physicians wrote a lethal prescription for a terminally ill resident.

Choosing to participate in the process of dying rather than the process of healing is difficult for many physicians. Some physicians and many social and legal commentators have confused the issue by using such terms as "assisted suicide" and "physician-assisted suicide" for medically assisted dying. Medically assisted dying is not suicide in states that have enacted laws to legalize it, and the continuing use of such biased terms as physician-assisted suicide leads to confusion and ill-founded opposition.

Medically assisted dying laws and their implementation are still works in progress. Regardless of any faults or shortcomings, medically assisted dying laws have become a much better response to the needs of terminally ill patients than ignoring them and driving patients to commit suicide to end their distress.

It is not enough that the medical profession responds to the situation it has brought about. Government support, oversight, regulation, and funding are essential parts of the healthcare system. Laws that provide for medically assisted dying are needed in states where they are absent. Perhaps a nationwide law that legalizes medically assisted dying, as Canada has provided, should be enacted to give everyone a constitutional right to medically assisted dying, much as everyone has a constitutional right to cause their death by refusing medical assistance needed to keep them alive.

Finally, patients themselves must recognize they are both part of the healthcare system and its primary beneficiaries. To that end, they must become more proactive in making clear their wishes or desires for the ends of their lives. Addressing those wishes or desires is taken up in the final chapter.

# # # # #

Chapter 5

HEALTHCARE, PATIENTS,
AND THEIR END-OF-LIFE WISHES

"[T]he adoption of supportive medical aid-in-dying policies changes the relationship between doctor and patient to a patient-directed relationship for all end-of-life care decisions."[1]

Every adult should make plans to have their end-of-life wishes granted.

To avoid difficult situations later, begin by discussing what you want with family members. Then document your wishes in writing — that is, prepare what are broadly called "advance directives." These specify the healthcare and other specifics of your life you either want to have or don't want to have later, when you may be unable to speak for yourself.

If you wish certain treatments to be provided or withheld subject to your physical condition, make those wishes and conditions known. Do that before an accident, illness, or old age renders you unable to voice your wishes, just when the need to react arises unexpectedly. Families should not be left to guess what healthcare their loved ones would have wanted.

In addition to a conventional will and estate plan to deal with the disposition of your personal property, a variety of documents are used today to ensure that you receive the end-of-life and healthcare options you wish and to avoid those you do not. The documents give specific directions for caregivers and healthcare providers to follow in the event you become incompetent and are no longer able to give directions for your care. They provide the means for you to control your healthcare when you become mentally incompetent and are no longer able to speak for yourself.

Make your doctors and other care-givers aware of your wishes for healthcare. Though most advanced life-support treatments are reasonably tolerable, some are not, and a few are downright unpleasant.[2] They can involve having tubes forced down your throat and into your stomach, having a hole cut in your throat, being injected with paralyzing drugs, or having air forced into your lungs.

If you prefer *not* to have such procedures used to sustain your life, you have a constitutionally guaranteed right to insist they not be used for you. But your physician and anyone else who might offer such care needs to know your wishes if they are to avoid using them. Without any other direction, physicians will do whatever they feel necessary to keep you alive.

This chapter describes different types of documents that patients are using today to help their physicians and others provide healthcare that is consistent with their wishes. The documents act as an interface between a patient and an attending doctor when patients are unconscious or cannot talk. They should be discussed with family members (spouses, children, parents, siblings, and other relatives), close friends, physicians, psychiatrists for those under psychiatric care, and church pastors for those who wish to follow religious practices and beliefs. The documents should include the names of individuals, their postal addresses, email addresses, phone numbers, and their relationships to the patient. They are personal testaments that should be dated and signed, and some should also be witnessed and notarized to make them legally binding.

DOCUMENTS

Although some efforts at uniformity have been made, the forms generally differ among the states. Most forms can be down-loaded from web sites, and their blanks can then be filled in or their boxes checked to express an individua's wishes for what they would like either done or avoided. Informative articles about the documents can be accessed by entering the title of the document on a computer's web browser.

Do Not Resuscitate Order

A "Do Not Resuscitate" (DNR) order[3] is a legal order to withhold Cardiopulmonary Resuscitation (CPR) or Advanced Cardiac Life Support (ACLS) if an individual's heart stops beating or if the individual stops breathing. In medical terms, this means when a person is suffering either a respiratory or cardiac arrest, or a combination of the two.

Resuscitative measures to be withheld include chest com-pression (CPR), mouth-to-mouth assisted ventilation (breathing), endotracheal intubation (i.e., inserting breathing tubes to open the airway), defibrillation (electric shock to restart the heart), and the use of cardiotonic drugs to stimulate the heart. In practice, most people who need resuscitation require intubation to survive.

If a patient stops breathing or their heart stops beating, a DNR allows another individual or an emergency medical technician to intervene and take the action specified in the document. If the patient does *not* have a DNR order at hand, a physician or another individual can decide whether to intervene or not and what treatment, if any, to apply. In such a situation, an individual or physician might provide cardiopulmonary resuscitation that leaves the patient alive but suffering from such a poor quality of life that death would have been preferable. This is the type of unwanted intervention that can be avoided by having a Do Not Resuscitate order at hand when an individual stops breathing or their heart stops beating.

Out-of-hospital cardiac arrest is a major concern, with approximately 420,000 cases annually in the United States. Since the decision *not* to perform cardiopulmonary resuscitation is irreversible and leads to death, one should talk to their primary care physician, specialist, or attending doctor about the pros and cons of Do Not Resuscitate Orders before deciding to sign one for yourself.

Hospital practices vary. Some emergency facilities require a patient's standing Do Not Resuscitate order to be followed *only* if the patient cannot speak. Otherwise, an attending physician or nurse must ask the patient if their standing DNR order continues to be their decision and should be followed. The question may be raised again if the patient is transferred from an emergency facility to a hospital.

Individuals with terminal illnesses or who are at high risk for stroke, heart attack, or respiratory arrest should consider having a DNR order. Others who might also consider having a DNR order are individuals in good health who feel strongly about being resuscitated once their breathing or heartbeat has stopped.

DNR orders are usually just one-page documents. They can be included as part of advanced healthcare directives or living wills. Many states have standard forms available that are prepared and signed by physicians after consulting with the individual patient.

A DNR order must be signed by an individual or the individual's legal surrogate or healthcare decisionmaker. It should be clearly posted in an individual's home or near the patient in a hospital, or the form can be folded and carried on an individual's person. It may be included in a living will or an advance directive.

Individuals change their minds. If a patient appears lucid, an attending physician will likely ask a patient with a DNR order whether they wish to invoke it or have changed their mind and wish to receive medical care. If there is any doubt as to a patient's wishes, medical professionals may override or ignore a patient's wishes in the weeks and months before their deaths. It happens for a variety of reasons, and it can lead to invasive and fruitless testing, needless suffering, unrelenting pain, and a prolonging of the period before death. Patients can be tethered to monitors and machines despite their determination to reject treatment and their desire to die at home in the embrace of loved ones.

A variation on the Do Not Resuscitate order is a Do Not Resuscitate and/or Do Not Intubate order. This type of order lists the two medical procedures separately so that a patient can select one or the other, or both, by checking the procedures the patient wishes withheld. For example, the document might contain check boxes and wording like the following:

☐ Do Not Resuscitate (DNR): In the event of an acute cardiac or respiratory arrest, no cardiopulmonary resuscitation shall be initiated.

☐ Do Not Intubate (DNI): In the event of an acute or impending respiratory failure, no endotracheal intubation shall be done.

Physician Orders for Life-Sustaining Treatment

A Physician Orders for Life-Sustaining Treatment (POLST)[4,5,6] advises and allows emergency medical services to provide immediate care, possibly before or while transporting a patient to an emergency care facility. Other names and acronyms include Physician Orders for Scope of Treatment (POST), Medical Orders for Scope of Treatment (MOST), Medical Orders for Life-Sustaining Treatment (MOLST), and Transportable Physician Orders for Patient Preferences (TPOPP).

A POLST provides instructions that a person wishes to be taken for responding to specific emergencies or health conditions. It indicates actions to satisfy immediate needs that might range from limited intervention for comfort care to aggressive treatment. A typical POLST occupies two sides of a single 8 -1/2 X 11 inch sheet of paper. Forms and instructions for their use can be downloaded from the web. For access to one, simply enter "POLST" or "POLST form" on a computer browser and press Enter.

A POLST is prepared by an individual or their surrogate and their physician. It has a standardized, easily recognizable format that is valid throughout the nationwide healthcare community. It may specify that no life-sustaining treatment should be given in the event of a cardiac arrest or an individual's not breathing, or they may list the time limits (days, weeks, or months, for example) or the conditions for continuing supportive care, such as intubation and vasoactive medication drips, after which the life-supporting treatment is to be discontinued.

The use of POLST documents began in Oregon in 1991 as a means of understanding and responding to the treatment goals of individuals with advanced progressive illness. A POLST is a useful follow-on to a terminally ill patient's decision to enroll in a state's medically assisted dying program. The POLST was designed to ensure that an individual's preferences for medical treatments would be honored throughout the healthcare system. They now exist under varying names for most of the United States. According to the Wikipedia article "Physician Orders for Life-Sustaining Treatment" (accessed October 13, 2018). POLST currently exists at some level in 42 states and meets the national POLST standard in 18 states.

Ideally, a POLST is a collaboration between patients and their attending or primary-care physicians. Their goal is to help patients live the way they want until they die — that is, to receive the medial care they *do* want and avoid the medical care they do *not* want *and the conditions for each.* The patient (or his or her authorized surrogate) and the patient's primary care physician or other health-care professional discuss and select treatments that might be provided or withheld in response to the patient's current conditions.

It is up to the patient to say what they want their POLST to say. To satisfy that goal, patients and their healthcare professionals should discuss the following:

- The individual's diagnosis, including their general health, a list of their diseases or medical conditions, and a list of the medications they take.
- The individual's prognosis, including the course of the diseases or conditions that are likely to happen over time.
- The treatment options that are available to the individual, how they might help, and what side effects might they have.
- The selected treatments are identified in a standardized form, such as one developed by the state of residence. This might range, for example, from no treatment to limited intervention for comfort care

or to aggressive treatment in the event of an emergency, such as cardiopulmonary resuscitation or response to a stroke or heart attack.

• The individual's healthcare goals that are important to them and provide a good quality of well-being, including their relations to family members and any spiritual or religious considerations.

A completed POLST should be jointly signed by a patient and their doctor, though some states permit signatures of a nurse practitioner or physician assistant. A copy should be placed with the patient's medical records, and another copy should be carried with the individual in a wallet, billfold, purse or pocket as they move about.

Living Wills and Advance Healthcare Directives

First introduced in 1969, Living Wills[7] are the oldest form of advance directives. By 2007, 41 percent of Americans had completed living wills. Nearly every state in the union has passed laws that recognize and support Living Wills.

Living Wills and Living Wills and Testaments are two different types of documents. Living Wills express one's wishes for healthcare in the near-term future, whereas Living Wills and Testaments indicate how one wishes to divide one's assets among children, close relatives, and others after one's death.

Advance Healthcare Directives[8] are the written statements of an individuals' wishes for their healthcare and medical treatments — both what the individuals want done and what they want not to be done, and the conditions for each. They help avoid healthcare that is prolonged, painful, expensive, and emotionally burdensome to patients and their families. They do not appoint another person to make healthcare decisions; instead, they specify what should be done in response to certain conditions' arising. They are related to, but different from, powers of attorney and healthcare proxies, which authorize another person to act as their agent to make decisions on their behalf when they cannot. Advance Healthcare Directives are also known as Personal Directives and Advance Decisions.

According to a Wikipedia article, "Aggressive medical intervention leaves nearly two million Americans confined to nursing homes, and over 1.4 million Americans remain so medically frail as to survive only through the use of feeding tubes. As many as 30,000 persons are kept alive in comatose and permanently vegetative states. … [S]tudies indicate that 70–95% of people would rather refuse aggressive medical treatment than have their lives medically prolonged [while they remained] in incompetent or other poor prognosis states."[9]

Advance Healthcare Directives and Living Wills can specify the conditions under which an individual prefers to die rather than continue to live, such as being bed-ridden and dependent on others, being incontinent or unable to control one's bladder or bowels, being subject to incapacitating pain, blindness, deafness, or a specified combination of any of these.

Each state has limits on what an individual with an incurable condition and a limited life expectancy is permitted to include in their Advanced Healthcare Directive or Living Will and what a healthcare provider is allowed or required to do or not do. The following are examples of decisions that an individual can include:

- Whether the individual would like to receive any form of life support in the event of a medical emergency, or one would like not to receive certain specified types. Common forms of life support include Cardiopulmonary Resuscitation (CPR), heart defibrillation, assisted breathing, dialysis, and artificially administered food and water.
- Specific treatments an individual would like to receive in the event of permanent unconsciousness, such as a coma or persistent vegetative state, in which an individual is judged, with a reasonable degree of medical certainty, to be unable to think, feel, knowingly move, or be aware that they are alive, and for which there is no hope for improvement.
- Comfort care, including the use of any means possible to relieve pain, such as administering medication or creating a comfortable environment.

In addition to the provisions for healthcare while dying, a patient's wishes for the disposition of their body should be spelled out. The most common are burial or cremation. Other alternatives are the donation of hearts, kidney, and other organs for transplanting into the bodies of others and the donation of their cadavers for medical research.

Advance Healthcare Directives and Living Wills should be witnessed and notarized. As with other testamentary documents, they should be discussed with family members (spouses, children, parents, siblings, and other close relatives), friends, physicians, psychiatrists for those under psychiatric care, and, for those who wish to follow religious practices and beliefs, with their pastors or religious counselors. The documents should include the names of individuals, their postal addresses, email addresses, phone numbers, and relationships between them and the patient.

Power of Attorney

A Power of Attorney (POA)[11] is a legal directive that authorizes someone to represent or act on another's behalf in private affairs, business, healthcare, or some other legal matter. The person authorizing the other to act is the principal, grantor, or donor of the power, and the one authorized to act or represent the principal is the agent, surrogate, proxy, or "attorney in fact." Depending on the state or jurisdiction, powers of attorney must be witnessed and notarized, while others require only that they be signed by the principal or grantor. Agents are fiduciaries for their principals and are required by law to be completely honest with and loyal to their principals in their dealings with each other. Principals should take care in selecting agents to represent them, as some agents have stolen the assets of vulnerable principals, such as the elderly or ill-informed.

A power of attorney may end if the principal becomes incapacitated to make decisions or dies. If the power of attorney is meant to continue after the principal becomes incapacitated or dies, the power of attorney is called "power of attorney with durable provisions" or a "durable power of attorney."

Healthcare Proxy or Healthcare Power of Attorney

A Healthcare Proxy[12] or Healthcare Power of Attorney appoints a specified individual to make healthcare decisions on a patient's behalf when the patient is incapable of making and executing the decision themselves. In contrast to a living will, which specifies what a patient wishes done under certain conditions, a healthcare proxy or healthcare power of attorney allows the patient's surrogate to decide what is to be done when certain conditions arise. They give the appointed proxy the same rights to request or refuse medical care as an individual would have if he or she were still capable of making and communicating them.

Advance Planning Guides and End-of-Life Tool Kits

Studies of incapacitated patients who later recovered revealed that their proxies or surrogates had often chosen differently from what they would have selected themselves if they had not been incapacitated at the time. This was true even though the patients had filled out instructions in the types of documents already discussed above. Too much was left to "guesswork" by the surrogates, family, next-of-kin, and attending physicians.

Since the early 1990s, these problems have led to a "third generation" of directives. These include Advance Planning Guides and End-of-Life "Tool Kits" that are a complementary approach to the documents described earlier in this chapter. Rather than specifying medical responses to provide or withhold under certain conditions, they describe how a terminally ill patient would like best to live during their final days or months. They move the focus from specific treatments and medical procedures to a patient's values and personal goals.

The guides or kits can be obtained from the Compassion & Choices, Death with Dignity, and Aging with Dignity organizations.[13-17] The kits or guides can be ordered online from the organizations' web sites. When properly completed, signed, and witnessed, they are legal documents. They express the wishes of an individual for medically assisted dying and end-of-life care from a fatal disease or when afflicted with Alzheimer's, Parkinson's, Huntington's, amyotrophic lateral sclerosis, or other neurodegenerative disease. To this end, they do the following:

- Appoint a surrogate to speak for the patient when the latter cannot speak for themselves. This might be the patient's spouse, adult child, or adult sibling, or it might be a close relative or a close friend. The surrogate should know the patient very well and be available and agreeable to acting in the patient's stead on healthcare or other defined issues when the patient cannot.
- Describe the conditions for which an individual wishes specific life-support healthcare services and equipment that are essential to living should be provided, limited by certain conditions that the individual would find objectionable.
- Describe the healthcare or life-support services or conditions which the patient would find so objectionable or uncomfortable that they should *not* be provided or should be *discontinued* if they have already begun.
- Specify how long a specific life-support healthcare services and equipment that are essential to living should be continued, after which they should be discontinued, the equipment should be removed, and the patient should be allowed to die naturally.

- Specify what should be provided to keep an individual comfortable, free of physical pain, and able to enjoy and participate in life to an acceptable level.
- List the different sorts of care and attention should be provided by others during the terminal illness of someone who cannot provide them for themselves,
- Indicate what should be done if a healthy individual succumbs to a neurodegenerative disease, such as Alzheimer's, that renders them ineligible for medically assisted dying and completely dependent on others for such care as spoon-feeding to keep them alive. Should food and drink be denied so that they die from voluntarily stopping to eat or drink (VSED),
- Tell what sort of attention and care should be given by family members and other loved ones, including final wishes for reconciliation and resolution of past differences, forgiveness for past offenses, sharing memories of the past, and seeing that my body is properly buried, cremated, or otherwise cared for in the manner requested by the patient.
- Allow death to come peacefully when it comes.

GOVERNMENT-SPONSORED COMPONENTS FOR END-OF-LIFE HEALTHCARE

Sixty years ago, healthcare was a cottage industry, "with most physicians in solo or small group practice, hospitals and nursing homes mostly small and independent with many not-for-profit, and private health insurers not yet in the business of medical underwriting in order to avoid coverage of sicker patients."[18] The overall transformation of healthcare has been the consolidation of its components into large for-profit corporations, with fundamental changes in the roles of each.

Most importantly, improvement in our general health and our increased life expectancy is due to the availability of healthcare services and medicines as part of the public healthcare provided by our federal government. This began with the Public Health Service Act of 1944 under the Democratic President Franklin D. Roosevelt. This Act consolidated and revised the laws relating to the U.S. Public Health Service, and it was the beginning of a major involvement of the federal government in healthcare. Since then, healthcare has benefited from remarkable improvements in medical technology, much of it sponsored by federal and state grants and conducted in various hospitals and medical schools. Healthcare became a major form of business, and the federal government has been a major part and influence in it ever since.

The Older Americans Act of 1965 was the first federal initiative to provide comprehensive services for older adults. It responded to concern over the lack of community social services for older persons by providing meals-on-wheels and other nutrition programs, in-home services, transportation, legal help, elder abuse prevention, and caregivers support.

Another major advance in healthcare followed in 1966 with the enactment of the Medicare and Medicaid programs as part of Democratic President Lyndon Johnson's Great Society program. Medicare is a single-payer national health insurance program begun in 1966 under the Social Security Administration, and Medicaid is a joint federal and state program that helps with medical costs for some people with limited income and resources. Medicaid also offers benefits not normally covered by Medicare, such as nursing home care and personal care services.

Among the other healthcare acts that followed were the National Cancer Act of 1971, the Health Insurance Portability and Accountability Act of 199, the Health Care Consolidation Act of 1996, and the Hematological Cancer Research Investment and Education Act of 2001

Patient Protection and Affordable Care Act

Until early in 2010, however, our nation stood apart as the only major democracy in the world without a program of universal healthcare. That ended on March 23, 2010, when Democratic President Barack Obama signed into law the Patient Protection and Affordable Care Act[19] (in short, the Affordable Care Act, or ACA). The nickname "Obamacare" is also used to refer to the Patient Protection and Affordable Care Act of 2010.

The Patient Protection and Affordable Care Act was the largest overhaul and expansion of healthcare coverage since the passage in 1965 of Medicare and Medicaid. It covers all U.S. citizens and legal residents with income up to 133% of the poverty line

The complete text of the Affordable Care Act covers close to a thousand pages. It is one of the most controversial pieces of legislation in decades. Together with an amendment titled the Health Care and Education Reconciliation Act of 2010, which was passed by Congress and then signed into law by President Obama on March 30, 2010, ACA represents the U.S. healthcare system's most significant regulatory overhaul and expansion of coverage since the creation of Medicare and Medicaid in 1965.

The major provisions of Affordable Care Act came into force in 2014. Eligibility for Medicaid was expanded and there were major changes to individual insurance markets. By 2016, two years later, an estimated 20 to 24 million people had been added to those insured under the Act, and the uninsured share of the population had been cut approximately in half. New funding was provided by cuts to Medicare provider rates and Medicare Advantage and by a mix of new taxes. "Several Congressional Budget Office reports said that overall these provisions reduced the budget deficit, that repealing the ACA would increase the deficit, and that the law reduced income inequality by taxing primarily the top 1% to fund roughly $600 in benefits on average to families in the bottom 40% of the income distribution. The law also enacted a host of delivery system reforms intended to constrain healthcare costs and improve quality. After the law went into effect, increases in overall healthcare spending slowed, including premiums for employer-based insurance plans."[20]

The Affordable Care Act has faced repeated partisan challenges and opposition in Congress. Although the Supreme Court upheld the ACA in a 5-to-4 split decision in 2012, it ruled that states could choose not to participate in the expansion to ACA's Medicaid coverage. Although ACA was initially opposed by a slim plurality of Americans polled, by 2017 it had gained a majority of voters' support.

A large portion of the cost of medical care in the United States is paid by the federal government and private insurers. This is a matter of importance, and it has been the cause of bitter bipartisan disputes between progressive and conservative forces that have become very divisive. The costs are staggering.

- 1/2 of all medical expenditures in the USA go to pay for treating only 5 % of the total population.
- 1/3 of all Medicare payments go to treating people in the final year of their life, often with incurable chronic illnesses.
- 1/6 of all hospital patients are treated in Catholic affiliated hospitals, which are being purchased and merged with for-profit health management organizations (HMOs).

For details on ACA's provisions, see the Wikipedia article "Provisions of the Patient Protection and Affordable Care Act."

Medicare

Medicare[21,22] is one of two single-payer, social or medical insurance programs that have been sponsored by the U.S. federal government since 1966. (The other is Medicaid and is discussed in the section that follows.) It is funded by payroll taxes, premiums and surtaxes from beneficiaries, and general revenues. Many private insurance companies across the United States are under contract to the federal Social Security Administration. Both Medicare and Medicaid are administered by the U.S. Centers for Medicare & Medicaid Services in Baltimore, Maryland.

Medicare provides health insurance for Americans who are 65 years or older of age and have paid into the system through payroll deductions from their wages and salaries. It also provides health insurance to younger individuals who suffer certain disabilities identified by the Social Security Administration and to people having end-stage renal disease (a chronic kidney disease that may lead to kidney failure) and amyotrophic lateral sclerosis (a rare neuromuscular disorder commonly known as "Lou Gehrig's disease").

Medicare coverage is divided into three parts, A, B, and D, as follows:

Part A: Hospital Insurance
  • Inpatient care in hospitals
  • Skilled nursing facility care
  • Hospice care
  • Home health care

Part B: Medical Insurance
  • Services from doctors and other healthcare providers
  • Outpatient care
  • Home healthcare
  • Durable medical equipment (e.g., wheelchairs, walkers, hospital beds, and other equipment and supplies)
  • Many preventive services (e.g,, screenings, shots, and yearly "Wellness" visits))

Part D: Prescription Drug Coverage
  • Partial cost of prescription drugs (as negotiated with private insurance companies and drug manufacturers)

When one first enrolls in Medicare or during certain times of the year thereafter, an individual can enroll in either "Original Medicare," which includes Parts A and B, or in "Medicare

Advantage," which includes Part A, Part B, and usually Part D. Within these two main options there are variations in out-of-pocket costs and extra vision, hearing, or dental benefits. For help in choosing coverage, call 1-800-633-4227 or send an email to the Medicare Plan Finder at Medicare.gov/find-a-plan.

An individual who is already getting benefits from Social Security or the Railroad Retirement Board automatically gets Medicare Part A and Part B starting on the first day of the month of the individual's birthday.

Medicare covers roughly half of the healthcare charges for those enrolled. Enrollees must themselves cover the remaining costs, either with supplemental insurance, separate insurance, or out-of-pocket. In 2015, Medicare provided health insurance for over 55 million people.[23]

Medicaid

Medicaid[24] is a joint federal and state program in the United States that helps pay medical costs for some people whose income and resources are insufficient to pay for health care. Medicaid also offers benefits not normally covered by Medicare, such as nursing home care and personal care services. As of 2017, Medicaid provides free health insurance to 74 million low-income and disabled people.

Hospice Care

On the order of 85 to 90 percent of terminally ill patients who choose medically assisted dying are in hospice care, either in their own homes, the homes of friends, nursing homes, or other hospice facilities, at the time of ingesting a lethal drug to end their dying. About 30 percent of all Americans, including both terminally and non-terminally ill patients, are spending the final days of their lives in nursing homes.

Hospice care for terminally ill patients is not directed to curing illness or other medical problems; instead, it is for Medicare beneficiaries who do not want curative or rehabilitative treatment. It is focused on providing non-curative nursing care, counseling, and palliative medication to relieve suffering. Terminally ill patients who enroll in hospice care typically agree to forgo aggressive treatment with the goal of curing an illness; instead, they receive treatments with the goal of providing comfort.

Hospice care[25] provides part-time help with such daily activities as dressing, eating, bathing, essential body functions, and administering medications. It provides care for the sick, especially for patients who are chronically or terminally ill. If hospice care is provided in a patient's home, it requires a caregiver who is willing, capable, and available as needed. Alternatively, it may be provided in a nursing home or hospice. The latter is a home that is licensed to provide care for the sick and dying.

Medicare pays for hospice care and services for anyone with a serious illness whose doctor certifies that they have six months or less to live, and who agrees to forgo life-saving or potentially curative treatment. Medicare's hospice coverage includes the following services:[26]

- Physician services
- Nursing care
- Medical social worker service
- Counseling (dietary, pastoral, and other types)
- In-patient care
- Hospice aide and homemaker services
- Physical and occupational therapies
- Medical appliances, medications, and supplies
- Speech-language pathology services
- Bereavement services for families

Hospice care is an accepted component of the U.S. health-care system today for terminally ill patients who have been diagnosed with less than six months to live. It is largely defined and financed by the federally funded Medicare system and other providers of health insurance, including private health insurance plans.

Hospice care began in the United States in the late 1970s, when the federal government began viewing it as a humane option for the care of terminally ill patients. The Tax Equity and Fiscal Responsibility Act (TEFRA) of 1982 established a system to pay for inpatient hospital and hospice care and recognized Medicare as the secondary payer for health services to individuals who were covered by a private health insurance plan.

The Congress of the United States Congress began the Medicare Hospice Benefit in 1982, and it became permanent in 1986. Since then, hospice care for terminally ill patients has become a large part of the healthcare system, with an estimated 1.581 million patients in 2010. It covers 24-hour/7-day a week ("24/7") care in the homes of patients or their families' (about two-thirds of the total) and in home-like hospice residences, nursing homes, assisted living facilities, veterans' facilities, hospitals, and prisons.

Hospice care includes palliative care to provide physical, mental, emotional, and spiritual relief from the illnesses of terminally ill individuals. It is most often provided in out-patient facilities, such as nursing homes and hospices. It can also be given in the private homes of afflicted individuals who prefer spending the last of their lives in their own homes.

More than one-third of dying Americans use hospice care, and about 30 percent or more of Medicare's budget is spent on patients in the final year of their lives. If medically-assisted dying were available for terminally ill patients in hospice care, the savings for hospice care could be used to pay for other causes, such as education of the young, upgrading the nation's decaying infra-structure, increased police protection, psychological counseling to prevent suicide by depressed individuals, and many, many other social benefits that are currently not provided because of lack of funding.

Palliative Care and Palliative Sedation

Palliative care[27] is specialized medical and nursing care to relieve the pains and stresses of chronically or terminally ill patients. As part of that purpose, it helps satisfy the physical, intellectual, emotional, social, and spiritual needs of patients and their families. It is delivered by teams of physicians, nurses, dieticians, therapists, social workers, psychologists, religious or spiritual counselors, and other healthcare practitioners. It generally does not provide any curative care or treat diseases or illnesses, but it may do so if a patient's suffering is related to a terminal illness.

Palliative care recognizes that roughly one-third of terminally ill patients who receive a lethal drug to end their lives under medically assisted dying laws do not ingest the lethal drug. Instead, simply possessing the lethal drug restores enough of their autonomy over their lives that they continue to live. Many die within the six months of their prognosis, and others live longer. Palliative care can be used to help make their final days more comfortable, either by relieving physical pain or alleviating other types of distress.

Palliative sedation[28] is an option when normal palliative care fails. It is a means of last resort for relieving pain and providing a peaceful death for dying patients. Palliative sedation involves "the monitored use of nonopioid medications to create controlled sedation to the point of unconsciousness in a patient very near death, with the purpose of relieving symptoms that cannot be controlled using other measures."

Palliative care and palliative sedation are separate and distinct areas of medical practice. One or the other is always a component of hospice care. They are additional end-of-life options or adjuncts to medically assisted dying.

Geriatric Care

Geriatrics or geriatric medicine[29,30] is a new medical specialty that focuses on the unique needs of older people as they age. More precisely, "older people" means people who are 65 years of age or older. As a practical matter, most people do not need geriatric expertise until the age of 70 or 75.

Geriatric medicine began as a specialty during the early 21st century with the increasing numbers of elderly and terminally ill patients, Gerontology, or the study of aging, includes biologic, sociologic, and psychologic changes.

A geriatric patient is an older person afflicted with chronic illness and physical or mental impairment. Examples of impairments vary from reduced levels of hearing or sight, forgetfulness, and confusion to osteoporosis, Alzheimer's disease and other forms of dementia, and cancer. Geriatric physicians and nurses focus on preventative care (e.g., aids to prevent falling or to rise from a fall). They also help patients and their families adjust or cope with certain medical, mental, and physical conditions that develop later in life.

Geriatric care begins with an assessment and evaluation of the issues and challenges that a senior is experiencing, such as health issues, mobility and transportation issues, bathing and grooming issues, eyesight and hearing, mental and cognitive problems, depression, spiritual or religious concerns with life hereafter, etc. This is followed by the development of a plan to provide care for the issues identified in the assessment.

Geriatric physicians, also called geriatricians, are primary care doctors who are specially trained in the diagnosis, treatment, and prevention of disease and disability in older adults. Their education and training include a four-year undergraduate program followed by medical school and a three-year residency in internal or family medicine. They are based in hospitals, clinics, or private practice.

WITHHOLDING HEALTHCARE OR OTHER INFORMATION FOR RELIGIOUS REASONS

Many facilities and individuals that provide healthcare oppose providing such services as abortions and medically assisted dying because they violate religious beliefs and teachings. Under current law, while healthcare providers can legally refuse to provide *services* they object to for reasons of conscience or religion (for example, a Catholic hospital can legally refuse to perform abortions or to treat transgender people), they still have a legal and moral obligation to refer them to another healthcare provider that will provide the information and services they need and want.

On January 18, 2018, the Office for Civil Rights in the U.S. Department of Health and Human Services announced the formation of a new Conscience and Religious Freedom Division to satisfy healthcare providers who object to certain procedures on religious or moral grounds. Under the proposed rules, healthcare providers who oppose various practices could impose their religious beliefs on their patients by withholding vital information about treatment options — including end-of-life options such as voluntarily stopping eating and drinking, palliative sedation, and medically assisted dying. This is a serious threat to terminally ill patients, to medically assisted dying laws, and other patient-centered care. It means that federal tax dollars, which support religious hospitals and physicians, could be used to protect facilities and their staffs that willfully decide to hold back information from a patient and abandon them when they are at their most vulnerable.[31]

LEGAL PROCEDURES THAT FOLLOW DEATH

Regardless of how a person dies, certain legal procedures must be followed for the treatment of their corpse, the disposition of their properties among family members and other inheritors of the deceased's estate, and the receipt of insurance benefits.

Insurance policies generally have specific provisions regarding the disposition of estates in the event death is caused by an actual suicide. Suicide may limit or cancel benefits if a mentally competent individual commits suicide within a specific period (typically three or five years) from the date of the insurance policy's issuance. If an individual commits suicide after the termination date of the period for limiting or cancelling benefits, the estate and heirs receive the benefits specified in the insurance policy.

CONCLUDING COMMENTS

With so much at risk, individuals — and especially mentally competent patients who are terminally ill — should make any wishes for their end-of-life healthcare loud and clear. Otherwise they invite the sort of troubles illustrated by some of the hospital disasters and courtroom trials described in earlier chapters. Various types of documents have been developed to help individuals receive the type of end-of-life healthcare they with at. Use them!

Medically assisted dying has proven a useful and cost-effective way of dealing with end-of-life healthcare. We look to the following to happen in the near term:

- Enacting laws for medically assisted in states that do not yet have such laws in effect.
- Reducing the time and number of steps from making the initial request for a lethal drug to obtaining and using it.
- Reducing the cost of prescriptions for lethal drug doses.
- Instead of setting a single fixed time, such "not more than six months to live" for a patient's gaining access to medically assisted dying, let access be open to any patient whose death is judged by the combination of the attending and consulting physicians to be "any time in the near or far term foreseeable future, taking into account all of a patient's current medical conditions and circumstances," similar to the Canadian law for medically assisted dying.
- Expanding the curricula of more and more medical schools to include an early introduction to the special needs of the growing size and age of the population of the elderly and to the role of geriatric medicine and medically assisted dying.
- Addressing the rising costs of medical care to which citizens are entitled.

# # # # #

Appendix A

Resolution of the 2017-2018 Congress against Medically Assisted Dying Laws

The release of the Trump Administration's 2020 budget in mid-March 2019 has raised concern for the future of medically assisted dying in the United States. The budget prohibits the use of local funds to carry out the law in the District of Columbia, thereby depriving terminally ill residents of D.C. of access to assistance granted to them by law to alleviate their end-of-life suffering. If passed, the Administration's budget might encourage opponents of medically assisted dying to seek a nationwide ban on it.

It is important, therefore, that Congress have a better understanding of the laws for medically assisted dying and the errors and misunderstandings in the resolution opposing medically assisted dying that was introduced in the House of Representatives of the United States Congress on September 26, 2017. The Resolution is abbreviated in the following as "H. Con. Res. 80."

"H. Con. Res. 80" is a comprehensive statement of the political opposition to medically assisted. It was introduced by Representative Brad R. Wenstrup (R-OH) and subsequently introduced in the Senate. It appears bipartisan, with six Republican and seven Democratic co-sponsors. The resolution is non-binding and does not have the force of law. It was referred to committees in the House and Senate, and it had not been acted on at the time of this book's writing.

Some of the objections are against medically assisted dying itself. Others are against possible abuses or misuses against elders, minorities and other patients.

Unfortunately, "H. Con. Res. 80" is largely a collection of misunderstandings caused by the improper use of words or names, especially by the use of the term "assisted suicide" for what is correctly described as medically assisted dying or medical aid in dying. Assisted suicide is also used for such names as "death with dignity, end-of-life options, aid-in-dying, or similar names that have been used.

Assisted suicide is a synonym for euthanasia and is illegal in the United States. What is properly described as medically assisted dying or medical aid in dying should NOT be called assisted suicide.

Medically assisted dying or medical aid in dying is a procedure that is legal in the states and the District of Columbia that have enacted laws to make it legal.

Oregon's law for medially assisted dying, which is named the Death with Dignity Act, had been in effect in Oregon for 19 years before "H. Con. Res. 80" was drafted. Similar laws for medically assisted dying have been in effect in several other states for lesser times. The Supreme Court of the United States has upheld the legality of the laws.

Despites its misuse of the term "assisted suicide" and other errors, "H. Con. Res. 80" does provide a convenient listing of issues that have been voiced over and over against medically assisted dying laws. Let us recognize it for just that.

The laws are operating very well, and no examples of serious problems have occurred to the writer's knowledge

"H. Con. Res. 80" consists of 24 sections, beginning with an introduction that is followed by 22 "Whereas" clauses and ends with the resolution itself. Its full text is reproduced below, with comments inserted after each of the 24 sections. For convenience, the comments are set off in a different font from the text itself.

The discussion of "H. Con. Res. 80" that follows begins with the resolution's introductory clause. This is followed by 22 "Whereas" clauses and ends with the resolution itself.

The first fifteen "Whereas" clauses express various reasons for opposing what medically assisted dying laws provide, and the last seven "Whereas" clauses (numbers 16 to 22) deal with the administration or management of medically assisted dying laws rather than the laws themselves.

H. Con. Res. 80

"Expressing the sense of the Congress that assisted suicide (sometimes referred to as death with dignity, end-of-life options, aid-in-dying, or similar phrases) puts everyone, including those most vulnerable, at risk of deadly harm and undermines the integrity of the health care system."

The term "assisted suicide" does NOT refer to "death with dignity, end-of-life options, aid-in-dying, or similar phrases." Assisted suicide is another term for euthanasia, which is illegal in the United States by any name. This sort of incorrect use of terms is exactly what "puts everyone, including those most vulnerable, at risk of deadly harm and undermines the integrity of the health care system."

The terms "death with dignity, end-of-life options, aid-in-dying, or similar phrases" (such as medically assisted dying and medical aid in dying) refer to end-of-life options that are legal in seven states and the District of Columbia and have been recognized as legal by the United States Supreme Court. Most of them were in effect when this resolution was written and had already been used to end the lives of several thousand terminally ill patients with compassion and dignity.

Suicide is taking one's own life *freely and intentionally.* The people who jumped from high stories of buildings set afire by the terrorist attack in New York City on September 11, 2001 did not commit suicide because they did not *intend* to kill themselves nor did they jump *freely or voluntarily.* They were impelled to jump to avoid being burned to death.

Medically assisted dying focuses on ending the process of dying, not on death itself. Medically assisted dying, like jumping from a tall building to avoid being burned alive, is a sane choice when one is driven by the pains and distresses of life caused by terminal illnesses. It is similar, though legally different, from a patient's right to reject life-saving care they the find objectionable, even though removing it will cause their death. Medically assisted dying is intended to end a prolonged period of dying that is painful and distressful.

The death of a terminally ill patient in compliance with all of the conditions of a state law that legalizes medically assisted dying is legal and is NOT suicide, as is recognized by the Supreme Court of the United States.

The misuse of terms, whether done in ignorance or deliberately to mislead others, undermines the integrity of the healthcare system.

1. "Whereas "suicide" means the act of intentionally ending one's own life, preempting death from disease, accident, injury, age, or other condition:"

   To be precise, the meaning of suicide should include that suicide is ending one's life both intentionally and *freely* (that is without being compelled or pressured to do so).

2. "Whereas 'assisting in a suicide' means knowingly and willingly prescribing, providing, dispensing, or distributing to an individual a substance, device, or other means that, if taken, used, ingested,

or administered as directed, expected, or instructed, will, with reasonable medical certainty, result in the death of the individual, preempting death from disease, accident, injury, age, or other condition;"

In states where medically assisted dying IS legal, "knowingly and willingly prescribing, providing, dispensing, or distributing to an individual a substance, device, or other means that, if taken, used, ingested, or administered as directed, expected, or instructed, will, with reasonable medical certainty, result in the death of the individual, preempting death from disease, accident, injury, age, or other condition" is NOT "assisting in suicide." It is wrong for this resolution is worded in such a way as to suggest the medically assisted dying, in states that have passed laws to make it legal, is in any way assisting in a suicide.

In states that have NOT enacted laws to legalize medically assisted dying, "assisting in a suicide" means taking part in euthanasia, which IS illegal.

3. "Whereas society has a longstanding policy of supporting suicide prevention such as through the efforts of many public and private suicide prevention programs, the benefits of which could be denied under a public policy of assisted suicide;"

Again, "assisted suicide" is euthanasia. It is illegal. It is contrary to policies that support suicide prevention. But, "medically assisted dying: is NOT "assisted suicide." This resolution should NOT be worded in such a way as to suggest "medically assisted dying" is "assisted suicide." To do so is simply ignorant or deliberately using incorrect language to mislead the reader.

4. "Whereas assisted suicide most directly threatens the lives of people who are elderly, experience depression, have a disability, or are subject to emotional or financial pressure to end their lives."

Again, "assisted suicide" is euthanasia. It is illegal. It is contrary to policies that support suicide prevention. "Medically assisted dying' is NOT "assisted suicide."

Medically assisted dying laws provide for exami-nation of terminally ill patients, many of whom "are elderly, experience depression, have a disability, or are subject to emotional or financial pressure to end their lives," by two physicians — not once, but twice. If they have any doubt that a patient is depressed or mentally incompetent, they refer the patient for examination by a psychiatrist or licensed psychologist. If they are found to be depressed or mentally incompetent, they are not allowed to proceed in their quest for medically assisted dying; instead, they are referred to psychiatric or psychological treatment.

Medically assisted dying laws also provide witnesses to a patient's signing a request for a prescription for a lethal drug, at least one witness must be neutral, with no connection to the patient or their estate.

Medically assisted dying laws provide for psychological analysis and counseling for the elderly, the depressed, the disabled, and those with emotional problems. They have special procedures and caveats for preventing financial pressures, such as those exerted by individuals who will inherit any of the terminally ill patient's estate.

5. "Whereas the Oregon Health Authority's annual reports reveal that pain or the fear of pain is listed second to last (25 percent) among the reasons cited by all patients seeking lethal drugs since 1998, while the top five reasons cited are psychological and social concerns: "losing autonomy" (92 percent), "less able to engage in activities that make life enjoyable" (90 percent), "loss of dignity" (79 percent), "losing control of bodily functions" (48 percent), and "burden on family friends/care-givers" (41 percent);"

Oregon and some of the other states with medically assisted dying laws do provide annual reports that include statistics for the number of patients who choose to use medically assisted dying law. The information is used to help provide proper counseling focused on the reasons different terminally ill patients' have for applying for lethal doses to end their specific types of distress and suffering.

6. Whereas the United States Supreme Court has ruled twice (in *Washington v. Glucksberg* and *Vacco v. Quill*) that there is no constitutional right to assisted suicide, that the Government has a legitimate interest in prohibiting assisted suicide, and that such prohibitions rationally relate to "protecting the vulnerable from coercion" and "protecting disabled and terminally ill people from prejudice, negative and inaccurate stereotypes, and 'societal indifference;'"

Again, "medically assisted dying' is NOT "assisted suicide." Also, when properly defined, "assisted suicide" is the same as euthanasia and is illegal in all states and is contrary to policies that support suicide prevention.

The initial portion of this "Whereas" clause is correct. That is, the Supreme Court has indeed ruled that "there is no constitutional right to assisted suicide [i.e., to euthanasia]." More properly, the Supreme Court has ruled that there is no constitutional right to medically assisted dying (aka medical aid in dying and other names)

The Supreme Court has ruled that suicide is a matter for states to decide. It has specifically ruled that Oregon's law for medically assisted dying (titled the state's "Death with Dignity Act") is legal. Oregon's law is the model for similar laws that have been enacted in five other states and the District of Columbia. The Supreme Court of the state of Montana in the case of *Baxter, et al. v. Montana, et al.,* has also upheld the right of Montana residents to medically assisted dying.

7. "Whereas clearly expressing that assisted suicide is not a legitimate health care service, Congress passed, with a nearly unanimous vote, and President Bill Clinton signed, the Assisted Suicide Funding Restriction Act to prevent the use of Federal funds for any item or service, including advocacy, provided for the purpose of causing, or assisting in causing, the death of any individual such as by assisted suicide, euthanasia, or mercy killing."

This is another misunderstanding caused by the continual misuse or misunderstanding of "assisted suicide" as a synonym for medically assisted dying. The findings and purpose of the Assisted Suicide Funding Restriction Act, which was decided on April 30, 1996, are as expressed by Section 2 of the findings, which reads as follows:

"Congress finds the following:

"(1) The Federal Government provides financial support for the provision of and payment for health care services, as well as for advocacy activities to protect the rights of individuals.

"(2) Assisted suicide, euthanasia, and mercy killing have been criminal offenses throughout the United States and, under current law, it would be unlawful to provide services in support of such illegal activities.

"(3) Because of recent legal developments, it may become lawful in areas of the United States to furnish services in support of such activities.

"(4) Congress is not providing Federal financial assistance in support of assisted suicide, euthanasia, and mercy killing and intends that Federal funds not be used to promote such activities."

At the time this law was passed, Congress was aware that there were efforts underway to enact state laws, such as medically assisted dying (and perhaps even assisted suicide, euthanasia, and mercy killing, which are three names for the same thing and have long been illegal in all states.)

8. "Whereas a handful of States have authorized assisted suicide, but over 30 States have rejected over 200 attempts at legalization since 1994;"

Medically assisted dying has admittedly been a tough sell. A major reason for this opposition is the misrepresentation and misuse of terms, such as done repeatedly in "H. Con. Res. 80."

Opposition to medically assisted dying laws is slowly being replaced by acceptance as misunder-standings are corrected. In fact, polls show that the majority of Americans now (on the order of 70 percent) are now in favor medically assisted dying laws. Better than a 3-to-2 majority of licensed physicians are also in favor of medically assisted dying. Many state and regional medical organizations are likewise in favor. The American Medical Association withdrew it opposition at its annual meeting in Chicago in June 2018. The state and federal elections of 2017 and 2018 also sent a message in favor of medically assisted dying laws by defeating for reelection a large majority of members of Congress who had opposed such laws and were running for reelection.

9. "Whereas States that authorize assisted suicide for terminally ill patients do not require that such patients receive psychological screening or treatment, though studies show that the over-whelming majority of patients contemplating suicide experience depression;"

This is another misuse of the term "assisted suicide."
Also, the statement is absolutely false when applied to

medially assisted dying. In fact, the laws for medically assisted dying require that two physicians must verify that patients are mentally competent and are not depressed or contemplating suicide. If there is any doubt of this, the patient must be referred to a psychiatrist or license psychologist for evaluation. If a patient is found incompetent, depressed, or contemplating suicide, they are referred to proper healthcare and rejected for medically assisted dying. *Read the medically assisted dying laws of Oregon and other states.*

10. "Whereas the laws of such States contain no requirement for a medical attendant to be present at the time the lethal dose is taken, used, ingested, or administered to intervene in the event of medical complications;"

   Experience with medically assisted dying has shown that complications have been rare, and no instances have been reported as having severe problems when the process is properly followed. In the great majority of cases (over 90%) family and friends are present when the patient ingests the lethal dose. They can intervene if help is needed.

11. "Whereas such State laws contain no requirement that a qualified monitor be present to assure that the patient is knowingly and voluntarily taking, using, ingesting, or administering the lethal dose;"

   The statement is not necessarily correct. In the great majority of cases (over 90%), family and friends are present when the patient ingests the lethal dose. Sometimes a patient's physician on knowledgeable lawyer or priest is present. This is much more presence than for the great majority of the more than 40,000 suicides committed each year, which is an alternative for any patient who prefers the use of a medically assisted dying law.

   Although states are aware that their laws do not require qualified to be present, none have indicated any problem or need to date that would justify their cost. There has been no demonstrated need that a monitor be present.

12. "Whereas the laws of such State laws contain no requirement to secure lethal medication if unwanted or if death occurs before such medication is used;"

If the lethal medication is obtained but not used because the patient has died from their terminal illness or other causes, the prescription should be properly disposed of, just as in the countless cases of expired or no longer used prescriptions for other medicines, many of which are toxic and dangerous if not used properly. Opioids and caches of sleeping pills are just two example that exists for roughly 70,000 deaths per year.

Medically assisted dying laws are well managed and administered by the Departments of Health of the states that have enacted medically assisted dying laws. There is no indication that that the possibility posed by the "Whereas" clause exists or is prevalent enough to warrant the cost of oversight to avoid improper use of a lethal dose obtained to use for medically assisted dying.

13. "Whereas such State laws do not prevent family members, heirs, or health care providers from pressuring patients to request assisted suicide;"

This is yet another misuse of the term "assisted suicide" as a substitute for medically assisted dying.

Note that the caveats of medically assisted dying laws require two meetings, each with two doctors who act independently of the other, possibly a meeting or more with a psychiatrist or licensed psychologist, and a couple of witnesses, at least of one whom must have no legal interest in the patient's estate. Beyond that, improperly pressuring a patient to request medically assisted dying would be the same as "aiding, assisting, or encouraging another to take their own life," which is a felony in all states and liable for a fine or possible imprisonment.

14. "Whereas such States qualify some patients for assisted suicide by using a broad definition of "terminal disease" and "going to die in six months or less" that includes diseases (such as diabetes or HIV) that, if appropriately treated, would not otherwise result in death within six months;"

This is yet another misuse of the term "assisted suicide" as a substitute for medically assisted dying.

Any patient who suffers from a terminal disease that would result in their deaths unless treated have the right to reject any life-saving procedure or equipment that they object to. They can end their distress by rejecting the medical means to keep them alive and use palliative care to avoid physical pain until they expire. They do not need medically assisted dying laws to provide this. They already have it.

15. "Whereas it is extremely difficult even for the most experienced doctors to accurately prognosticate a six-month life expectancy as required, making such a prognosis a prediction, not a certainty;"

The uncertainty in medical prognoses for the end of life has not caused any problem. Medically assisted dying is a win-win proposition whether the patient dies earlier of later than diagnosed. In fact, many patients among those who receive lethal drugs but do not use them; instead, they are so encouraged by having the lethal drugs to use anytime they wish that they go on living and enjoying life, such as it might be, for much longer than their diagnosis. A few such patients have lived for more than two years beyond their prognosis for six-months or less.

16. "Whereas reporting requirements vary by State, but when required, rely on prescribing physicians or dispensing pharmacists to self-report;"

This has caused no significant problem.

17. "Whereas such reporting is neither conducted by an objective third party nor of sufficient depth and accuracy to effectively monitor the occurrence of assisted suicide;"

The term "assisted suicide" should be replaced by "medically assisted dying."

Overall, the Health Departments of the different states with medically assisted dying are doing an excellent job of administering and managing the law. More manpower and funding would be needed to monitor its operations more fully.

18, "Whereas there is an astounding lack of transparency in the practice of assisted suicide to the extent that State health departments and other authorities admittedly have no method of knowing if it is being practiced within the bounds of State laws and have no funding or authority to make such a determination;"

Responsibilities are well defined and assigned, and accountabilities are being properly addressed.

19. "Whereas some State laws actively conceal assisted suicide by directing the physician to list the cause of death as the underlying condition without reference to death by suicide;"

The logic behind listing the cause of death as the terminal illness (or as some other cause that has intervened to cause death or as natural cause) is because it is the pain or distress caused by the terminal illness that drives the patient to use medically assisted dying to end the process of dying.

It is the same logic as listing the cause of death as the terrorist attack or the raging fire behind them rather than suicide for the people who jumped to their deaths from high towers in New York City in the terrorist attack of September 11, 2001, as discussed earlier. Suicide is the taking of one's life *freely and intentionally* – that is, deliberately, with the intent to end their lives and taken freely or voluntarily without being caused by an impelling force. Those who jumped from high towers during the terrorist attack of September 11, 2001 in New York City did so as a sane and reasonable act to avoid the pain and agony of being burned alive. They did NOT commit suicide. They chose a quick and violent death to a slow and painful one. Terminally ill patients similarly choose medically assisted dying to avoid the pain and agony of their terminal illness. They do NOT commit suicide. Their act is a sane and reasonable act that is legally recognized as NOT suicide when carried out according to state laws that contain provisions to avoid abuses or misuse.

20. "Whereas the confidential nature of end-of-life decisions makes it virtually impossible to effectively monitor a physician's behavior to prevent abuses, making any number of safeguards insufficient;"

Not true. Everything is being done to ensure terminally ill patients are themselves competent and free of depression of suicidal tendencies before allowing them to obtain a lethal drug. They usually have family members or friends helping them. Physicians and any psychiatrists or psychologists involved are licensed, and with two physicians to check and monitor the other as well as attend the patient there is good oversight.

Patients are themselves becoming more active in documenting their end-of-life desires in various types of advance directives. Most of the forms for advance directives can be obtained from web sites. More public education on their use would be helpful. The medical profession is also providing more training in geriatric medicine. Organizations such as Death with Dignity and Compassion & Choices are active in educating terminally ill patients and their family members. Improvement are being made and problems are being addressed where needed.

21. "Whereas the cost of lethal medication is far less costly than many life-saving treatments, which threatens to restrict treatment options, especially for disadvantaged and vulnerable persons, as has happened in several known cases and presumably many more unknown in which insurers have denied and/or delayed coverage for life-saving care while offering to cover assisted suicide;"

The term "assisted suicide" at the end of this "Whereas" should read "medically assisted dying."

Medically assisted dying is a choice for terminally ill patients in states which have enacted laws to legalize it. If a case occurs such as described occurs in a state where medically assisted dying is legal, the choice of life-saving care is one of the alternatives the patient or their surrogate can and should discuss. If an insurer restricts care in any way, the patient or their surrogate can enlist the aid of a healthcare worker to rectify the situation, and the Health Division of a state can help with appropriate action against the insurer for refusing life-saving care to which the patient is entitled.

22. "Whereas access to personal assistance services such as in-home hospice and palliative care, home health care aides, and nursing care/nursing assistance is regretfully limited and subject to long waiting lists in many areas, placing systemic pressure on patients in need of such personal assistance services to resort to assisted suicide:"

The term "assisted suicide" at the end of this "Whereas" should read "medically assisted dying."

When physicians counsel terminally ill patients to determine whether or not to provide medically assisted dying and suggest alternatives, such as in-home hospice and palliative care, home healthcare aides, and nursing care or assistance, many change their minds and choose an alternative rather than medically assisted dying.

Medically assisted dying and the alternatives both cost money, and the amount of money available in our nation's healthcare service is inadequate to do a much better job.

Many terminally ill patients who seek medically assisted suicide change their minds when counseled with physicians about alternative and choose other services.

Unless a terminally ill patient has the choice of using medically assisted dying or an alternative provided by our nation's healthcare system, the only choice left are either to continue in pain and suffering or to commit suicide, or ask for help to die by euthanasia.

"Resolved by House of Representatives (the Senate concurring), That it is the sense of the Congress that the Federal Government should ensure that every person facing the end of their life has access to the best quality and comprehensive medical care, including palliative, in-home, or hospice care, tailored to their needs and that the Federal Government should not adopt or endorse policies or practices that support, encourage, or facilitate suicide or assisted suicide, whether by physicians or others."

There is no opposition to or disagreement with the first part of the resolution, which supports comprehensive medical care, such as the Affordable Care Act (also known as Obamacare and by the acronym ACA), and other programs such as Medicare and Medicaid.

But let's be honest about the remainder of this resolution. Nobody is asking anyone, including members of Congress, to ask the Federal Government to "adopt or endorse policies or practices that support, encourage, or facilitate suicide or assisted suicide, whether by physicians or others." Facilitating suicide and assisted suicide are synonyms for euthanasia or mercy killing, which is illegal in all states in the United States. They are NOT what medically assisted dying is all about.

When carried out in accord with the provisions of state laws that have legalized it, medically assisted dying is NOT suicide or assisted suicide or euthanasia or mercy killing. Medically assisted dying is a compassionate alternative to suicide when it is carried out in accord with state laws that have legalized it. States that have not yet enacted laws to provide for medically assisted dying with proper wording to avoid abuses or misuses should do so as soon as possible.

CONCLUDING COMMENTS

It is unfortunate that state laws named Death with Dignity or Compassionate End-of-Life Options should have been labeled Assisted Suicide or Physician-Assisted Suicide instead of a more descriptive term, such as Medically Assisted Dying or Medical Aid in Dying. Using suicide as part of the name has created misunderstanding and opposition to medically assisted dying, which provides a compassionate alternative to suicide. That is essentially the purpose of medically assisted dying laws – to provide a compassionate and dignified death and to avoid an ugly suicide.

We have on the order of 44,000 suicides a year in the United States. Please support efforts to reduce that number.

It is understandable that names such Assisted Suicide or Physician-Assisted Suicide were misunderstood and initially raised strong opposition among physicians, many of whom had spent their professional lives doing their best to cure ills and prolong lives. Most physicians and many regional medical societies now support laws for medically assisted dying. The American Medical Association has withdrawn its opposition and taken a neutral position at its annual meeting in Chicago in June 2018 while it continues to study its position. The National Academy of Medicine has undertaken a 5-part program to advance the medical profession's participation in geriatric medicine, including medically assisted dying.

Medically assisted dying laws have now operated for 21 years in Oregon, 10 years in Washington, and lesser times in five other jurisdictions. They have operated successfully, with no significant problems. They have helped over 4,000 terminally ill patients end their lives with dignity rather than an ugly suicide.

Medically assisted dying is supported by a majority of residents and active voters. For decades, while improper names for medically assisted dying caused opposition, many lawmakers feared sponsoring medical aid-in-dying laws would harm their chances of getting re-elected. That fear was dispelled by the state and federal elections of 2017 and 2018. Results from those elections demonstrated how politically wrong was the support for the positions and reasons expressed in H. Con. Res. 80.

Nearly all lead sponsors of medically assisted dying bills who ran for election or re-election in 28 states won. That total included 13 out of 14 state senators and 49 out of 53 state representatives. At least five governors who publicly supported medical aid in dying — David Ige in Hawaii, Gavin Newsom in California, J.B. Pritzker in Illinois, Gretchen Whitmer in Michigan and Michelle Lujan Grisham in New Mexico — won election. In addition, Representative Keith Rothfus of Pennsylvania, a sponsor of a failed resolution to overturn Washington, D.C.'s Death with Dignity Act and a co-sponsor of H. Res. Con. 80 was defeated for re-election.

Medically assisted dying is a valuable part of our nation's healthcare system. It deserves the full support of both houses of our Congress.

And the use of improper names that cause or promote misunderstanding should end. It would be a form of dishonesty to continue their use.

# # # # #

BIBLIOGRAPHY

Anon., *Medicare & You: The Official U.S. Government Medicare Handbook* (Department of Health and Human Services, USA, 2019)

Ira Byock, M.D., *Dying Well: The Prospect for Growth at the End of Life* (Riverhead Books, New York, 1997)

Patrick Dunn, M.D., as Task Force Chair and Co-Editor, *The Oregon Death with Dignity Act: A Guidebook for Health Care Professionals* (first edition 1998; latest edition 2008). Updated as information becomes available. Accessible online from Oregon Department of Health website.

Rebecca A. English, Catharyn T. Liverman, Caroline M. Cilio, and Joe Alper, *Rapporteurs*, "Physician-Assisted Death: Scanning the Landscape," Proceedings of a Workshop held on February 12-13, 2018 by the National Academy of Medicine, released June 27, 2018. Free download at https://www.nap.edu/read/25131

Atul Gawande, M.D., *Being Mortal: Medicine and What Matters in the End* (Metropolitan Books, Henry Holt and Company, New York, 2018),

John Geyman, M.D., *Crisis in U.S. Health Care: Corporate Power v. The Common Good* (Coperrnicus Healthcare, Friday Harbor, Washington, 2017

Neil M. Gorsuch, Ph.D., J.D., *The Future of Assisted Suicide and Euthanasia* (Princeton University Press, 2006)

Derek Humphry, *Final Exit: The Practicalities of Self-Deliverance and Assisted Suicide for the Dying* (Delta Trade, Edition 3.1, April 2010). Now in its third edition, *Final Exit* has been a national best seller since it was first published in 1991.

Mugambi Jouet, *Exceptional America: What Divides Americans from the World and from Each Other* (University of California Press, April 2017)

Barbara Coombs Lee, *Finish Strong: Putting **Your** Priorities First at Life's End* (Compassion & Choices, 2019)

Philip A. Rizzuto and Daniel M. Walker, Committee Co-Chair, *Dying in America: Improving Quality and Honoring Individual Preferences Near the End of Life*, (National Academy for Medicine, 2014, 638 pages, ISBN 978-0-309-39310-1)
Free download at http://nap.edu/18748

Haider Warraich, M.D., *Modern Death: How Medicine Changed the End of Life* (St. Martin's Press, New York, 2017)

NOTES, REFERENCES, AND CITATIONS

Chapter 1: Medically-Assisted Dying as an End-of-Life Option

1. The two lines "Grow old along with me! The best is yet to be/The last of life for which the first was made," are the opening lines of a poem titled "Rabbi Ben Ezra" by the English poet Robert Browning (1812-1889). The poem is in the form of a narration by a fictional older rabbi giving advice to a youth. The poem points out that although youth will fade, it will be replaced by the wisdom and insight of age.
2. National Center for Health Statistics, Centers for Disease Control and Prevention.
3. Walter B. Pitkin., *Life Begins at Forty* (McGraw-Hill, 1932)
4. Testimony of Dr. John P. Geyman, MD, a lead plaintiff in the leading case in the state of Washington in 1994 to legalize medically assisted dying. Dr. Geyman was a professor and chair of the Department of Family Medicine at the University of Washington School of Medicine from 1976 through 1990. In 1994, he was a professor emeritus at the University of Washington and had a private practice in family medicine. John Geyman, M.D., *Crisis in U.S. Health Care: Corporate Power vs. The Common Good*," Copernicus Healthcare, 2017
5. Joel Aleccia, "In Colorado, a low-price drug cocktail will tamp down cost of death with dignity," *Kaiser Health News*, December 14, 2016
6. David Orentlicher, Thaddeus Mason Pope, and Ben A. Rich, "Clinical Criteria for Physician Aid in Dying," *Journal of Palliative Medicine*, Volume 19, Number 3, 2016, pages 259-262
http://online.liebertpub.com/doi/pdfplus/10.1089/jpm.2015.0092
7. Sheila Holmes, et al., "Exploring the experience of supporting a loved one though a medically assisted death in Canada," *Journal of the College of Family Physicians of Canada*, September 2018: 64(9):e387-e393
https://www.ncbi.nlm.nih.gov/pmc/articles/PMC6135137/
8. Anon, "Philip Nitschke." *Wikipedia*
9. Anon., "Suicide legislation," *Wikipedia*
10. Thaddeus Mason Pope, "Voluntarily Stopping Eating and Drinking Is Legal –and Ethical – for Terminally Ill Patients Looking to Hasten Death," *The ASCO Press,* June 25, 2018
11. Lukas Radbruch and Liliana De Lima, "International Association for Hospice and Palliative Care Response Regarding Voluntary Cessation of Food and Water." *Journal of Palliative Medicine*, volume 20, number 61, Letters to the Editor, June 2017

https://doi.org/10.1089/jpm.2017.0077

12. Božidar Banović and Veliko Turanjanin, "Euthanasia: Murder or Not: A Comparative Approach," *Iranian Journal of Public Health*, Oct. 2014, vol. 43, number 10, pp 1316-1323

13. For a summary and critical assessment of euthanasia in the Netherlands, see Chapter 7: "Legalization and the Law of Unintended Consequences: Utilitarian Arguments for Legalization" of Justice Neil Gorsuch's book *The Future of Assisted Suicide and Euthanasia*, Princeton University Press, 2006. Gorsuch concludes that "To the Dutch government, the ultimate justification for assisted suicide and euthanasia does not really seem to be patient autonomy or suffering at the end of the day, but, increasingly a physician's subjective assessment about the patient's quality of life." (*Op. cit.*, pp. 102-142)

14. Anon., "Euthanasia in Canada," Wikipedia

Chapter 2: Experience of States
with Medically Assisted Dying Laws

1. The National Right to Life Committee (NRLC) is the oldest and largest national pro-life organization in the United States. It was founded on April 1, 1967 by the National Conference of Catholic Bishops, which is composed of all active and retired members of the Catholic hierarchy in the United States. It is a federation of state right-to-life organizations, and it has 50 state affiliates and over 3,000 local chapters nationwide. According to its mission statement, its areas of concern include "euthanasia and assisted suicide," among other right to life issues. [https://www.nrlc.org]

   NRLC works through legislation and education to oppose induced abortion (its original purpose), infanticide, euthanasia and assisted suicide [sic]. (per Wikipedia articles "National Right to Life Committee" and "National Conference of Catholic Bishops") In the strict meaning of the two terms, euthanasia is the same as assisted suicide, and it is a crime in the United States by either name. (The Criminal Code of each state typically states "Aiding, assisting, or encouraging another to take their life is a crime.") NRLC's use of "assisted suicide" as a synonym for medically assisted dying in its statements of opposition is a biased misuse of the term, intended to mislead others, especially voters. legislators, and educators.

   To emphasize what is correct: "Euthanasia" or its synonym "assisted suicide" IS a crime in the United States. "Medically assisted dying" is NOT a synonym for "suicide," nor is it a synonym for "assisted suicide," nor is it a synonym for "euthanasia." "Medically assisted dying" IS legal in states that have enacted laws to make it legal. "Medically assisted dying" is NOT legal in states that have not yet enacted laws to make it legal.

2. *Lee v. State of Oregon.* The plaintiffs in this case were doctors, patients, and residential care facilities
3. Ibid
4. Ibid
5. *Washington Times*, Jan. 18; as cited in Anon., "Does Not Have Authority to Block Oregon Physician Assisted Suicide Law," *Kaiser Health News*, June 11, 2009
6. Ibid
7. Margaret P. Battin, Agnes van der Heide, Linda Ganzini, Gerrit van der Wald, and Bregie D. Onwuteaka-Philipsen., "Legal physician-assisted dying in Oregon and the Netherlands: evidence concerning the impact on patients in "vulnerable" groups," Journal of Medical Ethics, 2007;33:591–597; as cited in Wikipedia article "Oregon Ballot Measure 16."
8. Anon., "Brittany Maynard," Wikipedia
9. As reported by Margaret Hartmann, "Brittany Maynard, 'Death With Dignity' Advocate, Ends her Life," *Daily Intelligeneer*, New York, November 3, 2014. "Play it forward" is an expression for asking that others work toward seeing that the benefits one has received from the work of benefactors is best repaid when others continue to work towards providing the benefits to others in the future. It was appropriate for Brittany Maynard to express that admonition to others, and to encourage them to campaign as she did on behalf of enacting medically enacted laws in states without them so that other terminally ill patients could end their lives with dignity, as she most assuredly did herself.
10. Oregon Department of Health, report for 2016
11. Lynne Terry, "20 years of Oregon's Death with Dignity Act," The Oregonian, Oct. 27, 2017 (based on statistics published in a September 2017 report in the *Annals of Internal Medicine.*
12. Linda Ganzini, et al., "Oregon physicians' perceptions of patients who request assisted suicides and their families," *Journal of Palliative Medicine*, June 2003, 6(3):381-390
13. Testimony of Harold Glucksberg, a lead plaintiff in the leading case Washington v. Glucksberg (1997) in the state of Washington in 1994 to legalize medically assisted dying. Dr. Glucksberg is an assistant professor of medicine at the University of Washington School of Medicine and practices oncology, the treatment of cancer, at the Pacific Medical Center in Seattle. He has published dozens of

articles in medical journals dealing with cancer. He regularly treated terminally ill patients with cancer.

14. Compassion in Dying v. State of Wash., 850 F. Supp. 1454 (W.D. Wash. 1994)
15. Ibid
16. Ibid
17. Federal Report. March 6, 1996;79:790-859, Compassion in Dying v. State of Washington, United States Court of Appeals, Ninth Circuit
18. A "liberty interest" is an interest that is deeply rooted in the nation's history and is protected by the Due Process Clause of the Fourteenth Amendment of the Constitution of the United States. A woman's right to an abortion is a "liberty interest" that is protected by the Fourteenth Amendment. On the other hand, a terminally ill patient's right to medically assisted dying is NOT a "liberty interest" and is NOT a constitutional right protected by the Fourteenth Amendment. https://www.ncbi.nlm.nih.gov/pubmed/11648417
19. Anon., "Baxter v. Montana," Wikipedia.
20. The Montana Supreme Court decision can be found at http://searchcourts.mt.gov/
21. David Orentlicher, Thaddeus Mason Pope, and Ben A. Rich, "Clinical Criteria for Physician Aid in Dying," *Journal of Palliative Medicine*, 2016, Vol. 19, No. 3
22. https://www.deathwithdignity.org/states/vermont/
23. http://www.patientsrightscouncil.org/site/vermont/
24. Howard Weiss-Tisman, Vermont Public Radio, April 6, 2017
25. Anon., "California End of Life Option Act," Wikipedia
26. Ahn vs Hestrin, Riverside Superior Court, Riverside, California, Case RIC 1607135
27. Data Report, California Department of Public Health, July 1, 2018
28. Mary Klein, "I'm dying, and I'd like D.C.'s Death with Dignity Act to help," *The Washington Post*, April 6, 2017
29. Julia Nicol and Marlisa Tiedemann., "Bill C-14: An Act to amend he Criminal Code and to make related amendments to other Acts (medical assistance in dying)," Publication No. 42-1-C14-E, April 21, 2016, Revised September 27, 2018. This publication by the Legal and Social Affairs Division of the Parliamentary Information and Research Service of the Canadian Parliament provides an excellent summary of Canada's law for medical aid for dying (MAID) and its implementation.
30. Ibid
31. Ibid

32. Anon., "Third Interim Report on Medical Assistance in Dying in Canada," June 2018

33. David R. Gruber, "Ten Facts About Medical Aid in Dying," *MD Magazine*, August 28, 2018. Dr. Gruber has 45 years of experience as a family physician in Oregon. He was appointed to the Oregon Board of Medical Examiners (now Oregon Medical Board) in 2001, and served seven years, including two years as president. He was honored as Family Physician of the Year in 1986 by the Oregon Academy of Family Physicians.

Chapter 3: Opposition to Medically Assisted Dying

1. Scott Kim and Thomas Strouse, observations delivered at the session on "Competency, Decision-Making Capacity and Voluntariness" at the workshop "Physician-Assisted Death: Scanning the Landscape," National Academy of Medicine, February 12-13, 2018

2. Brooke Myers Sorger, Ph.D., Barry Rosenfeld, Ph.D., Hayley Pessin, Ph.D., Anne Kosinski Timm, B.A., and James Cimino, M.D., "Decision-making capacity in elderly, terminally ill patients with cancer," *Behavioral Sciences & Law,* vol. 25, issue 3, May/June 2007, pp. 393-404

3. Buddhism is based on the teachings of Gautama Buddha of India (c. 563 or c. 480 BCE); Confucianism is based the teachings of the Chinese philosopher Confucius (551-49 BCE); and Taoism is a development by various Chinese philosophical schools centered on living in harmony with the Chinese principle of *Tao* (literally "the Way"). All three of these ancient teachings are philosophies of life based on humanistic or rationalistic principles, similar to the development of secular morality during the Enlightenment or Age of Reason and its later replacement for religious morality in western culture. They also emphasize a common form of life and simple rituals rather than elaborate rituals that emphasize a deity. See the Wikipedia articles Buddhism, Confucianism, and Taoism for more information on each.

4. As quoted in "Buddhism, euthanasia and the sanctity of life," by R. W. Perrett, *Journal of Medical Ethics*, 22(5), October 1996. This article also notes that Buddhism does not value human life as an *intrinsic* good, but that the birth of a human life is precious only because as a human "is it possible to practice the *dharma* successfully and achieve the goal of the elimination of suffering, i.e., *nirvana*." Anon, "Ethical and Religious Directives for Catholic Health Care Systems," United States Conference of Catholic Bishops, Fifth Edition, November 17, 2009.

5. Anon., Pope Says Assisted Suicide Is a 'Sin Against God'", CBS NEWS, Nov. 14, 2014
   http://www.cbsnews.com/news/pope-says-assisted-suicide-is-a-sin-againstgod/[https://perma.cc/F9HL-AQPK].
6. Anon., "To Live Each Day with Dignity: A Statement on Physician-Assisted Suicide," United States Conference of Catholic Bishops, June 16, 2011
7. Ann Newman, "Catholic Church Amps Up Its Fight Against Aid in Dying, *The Nation*, June 5, 2011
8. The sentence "Religion is regarded by the common people as true, by the wise as false, and by rulers as useful" is a short paraphrase of the following text from Edward Gibbon, *The History of the Decline and Fall of the Roman Empire* (first published in 1776; volume 1, chapter 2): "The policy of the emperors and the senate, as far as it concerned religion, was happily seconded by the reflections of the enlightened, and by the habits of the superstitious, part of their subjects. The various modes of worship, which prevailed in the Roman world, were all considered by the people, as equally true; by the philosopher, as equally false; and by the magistrate, as equally useful. And thus toleration produced not only mutual indulgence, but even religious concord."

   An earlier statement of Gibbon's thesis is that by the Roman poet and philosopher Titus Lucretius Carus (99-55 BCE) from his text *De Rerum Natura* (On the Nature of Things): "All religions are equally sublime to the ignorant, useful to the politician, and ridiculous to the philosopher." Lucretius's work, written before the time of Jesus Christ, influenced the efforts of various figures of the Enlightenment or Age of Reason in developing a new philosophy of humanism based on man to replace the old philosophy of behavior based on a god.

9. The phrase "separation between church and state" is generally traced to a letter by Thomas Jefferson to the Danbury Baptist Convention in Connecticut in January 1802 which contains the following: "Believing with you that religion is a matter which lies solely between Man & his God, that he owes account to none other for his faith or his worship, that the legitimate powers of government reach actions only, & not opinions, I contemplate with sovereign reverence that act of the whole American people which declared that their legislature should "make no law respecting an establishment of religion, or prohibiting the free exercise thereof," thus building a wall of separation between Church & State. Adhering to this expression of the supreme will of the nation in behalf of the rights of conscience,

I shall see with sincere satisfaction the progress of those sentiments which tend to restore to man all his natural rights, convinced he has no natural right in opposition to his social duties." (as quoted in the article "Separation of church and state in the United States" in Wikipedia)

10. The Crusades (1095-1510) were a series of religious wars sanctioned by the Roman Catholic Church during medieval times. It included the nine distinct well-known wars to recover the Holy Lands from Muslim rule (1095-1291). The lowest estimate of the number of fatalities caused by these nine crusades is 1 million. Many more religious wars spread across Europe and the near east from 1291 to 1510) to suppress paganism and heresy or to resolve conflicts between rival Roman Catholic groups, or for political advantage or territorial expansion. The Wikipedia article "Crusades" lists 39 different crusades. The longest of these was the Lithuanian Crusade of 1283-1410; it was fought in a series of campaigns and raids spread over 127 years to convert the pagan Grand Duchy of Lithuania to Roman Catholicism.

11. The Guelph and Ghibelline Wars (1215-1392) were a series of wars in Northern Italy for political and religious power between factions allied to Roman Catholic Popes and those allied with the Holy Roman Emperors.

12. The Inquisitions were a series of institutions sanctioned by the Roman Catholic Church to suppress religious dissent and heresies. They began in 12th- century France against the Cathars and Waldensians. They continued as the Medieval Inquisition up to the mid-15th century, and they expanded significantly in the Late Middle Ages and early Renaissance in response to the Protestant Reformation (1517-1648) and the Catholic Counter-Reformation (1545-). The best known and most notorious was the Spanish Inquisition (1478-1834), during which an estimated 3,000 persons judged guilty of heresy were put to death by being burned alive as part of a public spectacles called an *auto-da-fé* (literally an "act of faith"). These were designed officially to engage the populace in a process of reconciliation and penance; unofficially, they were meant to intimidate and suppress anyone openly opposed to the Church's teachings and practices. (Based on the following anonymous articles in Wikipedia: "Inquisition," "Spanish Inquisition," "Medieval Inquisition," "Roman Inquisition," and "Counter Reformation,"

13. The Thirty Years War (1618-1648) was a war between rival Catholic and Protestant states in the Holy Roman Empire. It was fought primarily in what is now Germany, which had earlier been

fragmented by the Protestant Reformation (1517-1648) into rival states whose rulers separated into Catholic and Protestant domains (e.g., lordships, fiefs and fiefdoms held by feudal land tenure) that became bitter rivals because of religious differences of their rulers. From Germany it gradually developed into a more general conflict involving most of Europe's great powers and became one of the most destructive wars in human history. It resulted in eight million fatalities – not only from actual warfare but also from violence, famine, and plague. (Anon., "Thirty Years War," Wikipedia)

14. The castrati were adult men who had been castrated while still pre-pubescent boys to preserve their high-pitched voices into adulthood. The early Catholic Church had a long tradition against allowing women to sing in church choirs, as set forth in Scripture: "Let your women keep silence in the churches: for it is not permitted unto them to speak" (*I Corinthians 14:34-35*). Because of this prohibition against women, the treble parts of music in church choirs were sung by young boys with the high-pitched voices of pre-puberty. Beginning in the mid-16th century, young pre-pubescent boys (whose voices broke after only a few years) were replaced by castrati in church choirs.

By removing the testicles of young boys before or shortly after they reached puberty, their bodies were unable to produce testosterone. As a result, their vocal chords when adults had remained small and child-like and extraordinarily flexible, with a vocal range much higher than that of uncastrated adult males. Another result of castration was that the limbs and bones of the rib cages that surround and protect the body's lungs often grew unusually long. This provided room for larger lungs and a more powerful voice. The castrati voices were larger and more powerful than those of young boys, and their maturity helped provide a more expressive range of emotions.

At the height of the craze for castrati voices in the 1720s and 1730s, upwards of 4,000 boys, typically with ages between 9 and 11, are estimated to have been castrated annually in the service of music – the best sang in operas, others sang in church choirs in Europe, and many others without sufficient musical talent became outcasts. Many came from poor homes and were sold by their parents to "music masters" who had them castrated. To prevent the child from feeling the intense pain of castration, they were given doses of opium or other narcotic. Many, (estimates range from 10% to 80%) were killed inadvertently by overly large doses that were lethal or by overlong compression of the carotid artery in the neck, which was used to render them unconscious during castration.

The Catholic church created a market for castrati by hiring them for its church choirs. In 1589 Pope Sixtus V re-organized the choir of Saint Peter's in Rome specifically to include castrati. By about 1789, there were more than 200 castrati in Rome's chapel choirs alone.

After the initial unification of Italy in 1861, castration for musical purposes was made illegal. In 1870, castrations were banned in the Papal States, the last political jurisdiction to do so. In 1878, Pope Leo XIII prohibited the hiring of new castrati by the church. By 1900 there were only 16 castrati singing in the Sistine Chapel and other Catholic choirs in Europe. In 1902, Pope Leo XIII ruled that new castrati would not be admitted to the Sistine Chapel. In 1903, Pope Pius X formally banned them from the Vatican. (Anon., "Castrati," Wikipedia)

15. In more recent time (20th to 21st centuries), there has been widespread incidents of child sexual abuse by Catholic priests, nuns, and member of religious orders. The abused have been mostly boys but also girls, some as young as three years old, with the majority between the ages of 11 and 14. The abuses have led to many allegations, investigations, trials and convictions, and have included revelations about decades of attempts by the Church to cover up reported incidents. (Anon., "Catholic Church sexual abuse cases," Wikipedia)

16. Kim Callinan and Omega Silva, "Advocating for the Option of Physician-Assisted Death," at the workshop "Physician-Assisted Death: Scanning the Landscape," National Academy of Medicine, February 12-13, 2018

17. Ibid

18. Neil Gorsuch, *The Future of Assisted Suicide and Euthanasia,* Princeton University Press, 2006; Chapter 9: An Argument against Legalization, pp. 157-180.

19. Ibid, page 174

20. Ibid, page 158

21. Anon., "Suicide Statistics," American Foundation for Suicide Prevention. https://afsp.org/about-suicide/suicide-statistics/

22. Anon, "Ethical and Religious Directives for Catholic Health Care Systems," United States Conference of Catholic Bishops, Fifth Edition, November 17, 2009.

23. According to its web site, "Providence Health & Services is a for-profit Catholic network of hospitals, care centers, health plans,

physicians, clinics, home health care and affiliated services guided by a Mission of caring that the Sisters of Providence began in the West 160 years ago." It was founded in 1856 by Mother Joseph and four other Sisters of Providence in what was then Washington Territory. They established hospitals, schools, orphanages, and other institutions to provide care in the pioneer communities of the era. According to their website, they "serve in 50 hospitals, 829 clinics and hundreds of programs and services in Alaska, California, Colorado, Montana, New Mexico, Oregon, Texas and Washington."

24. Anon., "Excommunication of Margaret McBride," Wikipedia
25. Nicholas Kristof and Zoe Ryan, "Sister Margaret's Choice," The New York Times, May 26, 2010.
26, Anon., "Thomas Olmsted." Wikipedia
27. Anon., "An Essay on Man," first published in 1733. Wikipedia
28. Wikipedia articles about "Humanism,' "Renaissance," and "Renaissance humanism"
29. Written by Delegates of the National Convention in Philadelphia, Pennsylvania, 1787, "United States Constitution," as cited in United States Constitution," Wikipedia.
30. Neil Gorsuch, *The Future of Assisted Suicide and Euthanasia,* Princeton University Press, 2006
31. Anon., "Suicide Statistics," American Foundation for Suicide Prevention. https://afsp.org/about-suicide/suicide-statistics/
21. Megan Brenan, "Americans' Strong Support for Euthanasia Persists," Gallup Poll on Politics, May 31, 2018 https://news.gallup.com/poll/235145/americans-strong-support-euthanasia-persists.aspx

Chapter 4: Physicians and Healthcare Systems

1. Anon., Principles of Ethics, American Medical Association (2001, as revised), Principle Number 1
2. Robert Lowes, "Assisted Death: Physician Support Continues to Grow," *Medscape Ethics Report*, December 26, 2016
3. Marcia Angell, "May Doctors Help You to Die?", *The New York Times Review of Books*, October 11, 2012
4. Julian J.Z. Prokopetz and Lisa S. Lehmann, "Redefining Physicians' Role in Assisted Dying," *New England Journal of Medicine*, July 12, 2012 (367:97-99).
5. Lindsey Bever, "American Medical Association to keep reviewing its opposition to assisted death," *The Washington Post*, June 11, 2018
6. Anon., "American Academy of Family Physicians Moves to 'Engaged Neutrality' on Medical Aid in Dying," American Academy of Family Physicians, October 26, 2018 as reported by *Compassion & Choices Media Contacts*

7. Anon., "American College of Physicians Reaffirms Opposition to Legalization of Physician-Assisted Suicide," *as updated* in "Ethics and the Legalization of Physician-Assisted Suicide: An American College of Physicians Position Paper," *Annals of Internal Medicine,* September 19, 2017

8. Philip A. Pizzo, David M. Walker, et al., *Dying in America: Improving Quality and Honoring Individual Preferences Near the End of Life,* Institute of Medicine (now the National Academy of Medicine), September 17, 2014

9. Anon., *Code of ethics of the American* Medical Association, T. K. and P.G. Collins, Printers, Philadelphia, 1848. A photostat of the Code is available in the U.S. National Library of Medicine. The Code was adopted at the meeting of the National Medical Convention in Philadelphia in May 1847.

10. Ibid

11. Ibid

12. Op. cit.

13. Anon., *Principles of Medical Ethics*, American Medical Association. Accessed on the Web October 27, 2018

14. Neil Gorsuch, *The Future of Assisted Suicide and Euthanasia*, Princeton University Press, 2016, page 119

15. Philip A. Pizzo, David M. Walker, et al., *Dying in America: Improving Quality and Honoring Individual Preferences Near the End of Life*, Institute of Medicine (now the National Academy of Medicine), September 17, 2014, page 2

16. As cited in the Wikipedia article "Union Pacific Railway Company v. Botsford,"

17. As cited in Carol Stamatakis, "Beyond Advance Directives: Personal Autonomy and the Right To Refuse Life-Sustaining Medical Treatment," New Hampshire Bar Association, *Bar Journal*, Winter 2007

18. As cited in Anon., "Schloendorff v. Society of New York Hospital," Wikipedia. Because Schloendorff had sued the hospital itself, not the physicians, the Court found that a non-profit hospital could not be held liable for the actions of its employees, in keeping with the principle of charitable immunity, which holds that a charitable organization is not liable under tort law. Between the 1940s and 1992, this doctrine of charitable immunity has been repealed or limited by almost every one of the United States.

19. Anon., In re Quinlan," Wikipedia

20. Anon., "Karen Ann Quinlan," Wikipedia

21. As quoted in Wikipedia article "Cruzan v. Director, Missouri Department of Health"

22. For a fuller account of the details of the Schiavo case, see the Wikipedia articles

23. For the views of a disability activist, see Arthur Caplan, "Ten Years After Terri Schiavo, Death Debates Still Divide Us: Bioethicist;" *Health*, March 31, 2015

Chapter 5: Patients and Their End-Of-Life Wishes

1. Kim Kallinan, "Transforming End-of-Life Care," *Compassion & Choices Magazine*, Spring 2018, pp. 8-9
2. Mickey MacIntyre and Sean Crowley, "Unwanted medical treatment: a painful nightmare we cannot afford." *THE HILL*, June 27, 2013
3. Anon., "Do not resuscitate," Wikipedia
4. Anon., "Physician Orders for Life-Sustaining Treatment," Wikipedia
5. Charles P. Sabatino and Naomi Karp, "Improving Advanced Illness Care: The Evolution of State POLST Programs," *AARP Public Policy Institute*, April 2011
6. Anon., "National POLST Paradigm." The National POLST Paradigm was created by the Oregon POLST Task Force to help patients get the medical treatments they want, and avoid the medical treatments they *do not* want, when they are seriously ill or frail. It is a set of patients' frequently asked questions and answers, stories of the experiences of patients and their families, healthcare programs, news, and other resources to help people live the way they wish to live until they die. Website: http://polst.org/about/
7. Anon., "Living Will," Wikipedia
8. Anon., "Advance healthcare directive," Wikipedia
9. *Ibid*
10. Anon., "Medical assistance in dying," Government of Canada, December 10, 2018
    https://www.canada.ca/en/health-canada/services/medical-assistance-dying.html
11. Anon., "Power of attorney," Wikipedia
12. Anon., "Healthcare proxy," Wikipedia
13. Anon., "My End of Life Decisions: An Advance Planning Guide and Toolkit," Compassion & Choices,
14. Anon., "My Directives," Death with Dignity National Center
15. The Aging with Dignity organization is based in Tallahassee, Florida. With help from the American Bar Association's Commission on Law and Aging and medical experts, it developed and introduce a Florida-only document that combined a living will and health care power of attorney with comfort care and spirituality matters in 1996. An online version called Five Wishes Online was introduced in April 2011 allowing users to complete the document

using an online interface or print out a blank version to complete by hand. A sample copy of the 12-page "Five Wishes" document is available at the web site of the Aging with Dignity organization and the following web site:
https://fivewishes.org/docs/default-source/default-document-library/product-samples/fwsample.pdf?sfvrsn=2

16 Anon., "Five Wishes," Wikipedia
17. Davies, Frank, "Living Will From Florida Goes Nationwide," *The Miami Herald*, 10/23/1998.
18. John Geyman, M.D., *Crisis in U.S. Health Care: Corporate Power vs. The Common Good*. Copernicus Healthcare, 2018
19. Anon., "Patient Protection and Affordable Care Act," Wikipedia
20. Ibid
21. Anon., "Medicare," Wikipedia
22. Anon., "Medicare (United States)," Wikipedia
23. Anon., 2016 Annual Report of the Medicare Trustees (for the year 2015), June 22, 2016
24. Anon., "Medicaid," Wikipedia
25. Anon., "Hospice," Wikipedia
26. Anon., "Hospice and End-of-Life Options and Costs," Debt.org https://www.debt.org/medical/hospice-costs/
27. Anon., "Palliative Care," Wikipedia
28. "Palliative sedation" in *Advanced Practice Palliative Nursing*, Oxford University Press, 2016; as cited in "Palliative Sedation: When Suffering is Intractable at End of Life" by Peg Nelson Bander in *Journal of Hospice and Palliative Nursing*, 2017, 19(5), pp. 394-401
29. Anon., "Elderly care," Wikipedia
30. Anon., "Geriatric care management," Wikipedia
31. Anon., "Department of Health and Human Services: New 'Conscience And Religious Freedom Division' Threatens End-Of-Life Choice," *Compassion & Choices Newsletter*, March 23, 2018

# # # # #

Lightning Source UK Ltd.
Milton Keynes UK
UKHW011213020819
347285UK00003B/553/P